Helping Students Overcome Substance Abuse

The Guilford Practical Intervention in the Schools Series

Kenneth W. Merrell, Series Editor

Books in this series address the complex academic, behavioral, and social–emotional needs of children and youth at risk. School-based practitioners are provided with practical, research-based, and readily applicable tools to support students and team successfully with teachers, families, and administrators. Each volume is designed to be used directly and frequently in planning and delivering educational and mental health services. Features include lay-flat binding to facilitate photocopying, step-by-step instructions for assessment and intervention, and helpful, timesaving reproducibles.

Recent Volumes

Responding to Problem Behavior in Schools: The Behavior Education Program
Deanne A. Crone, Robert H. Horner, and Leanne S. Hawken

Resilient Classrooms: Creating Healthy Environments for Learning
Beth Doll, Steven Zucker, and Katherine Brehm

Helping Schoolchildren with Chronic Health Conditions: A Practical Guide
Daniel L. Clay

Interventions for Reading Problems: Designing and Evaluating Effective Strategies
Edward J. Daly III, Sandra Chafouleas, and Christopher H. Skinner

Safe and Healthy Schools: Practical Prevention Strategies
Jeffrey R. Sprague and Hill M. Walker

School-Based Crisis Intervention: Preparing All Personnel to Assist
Melissa Allen Heath and Dawn Sheen

Assessing Culturally and Linguistically Diverse Students: A Practical Guide
Robert L. Rhodes, Salvador Hector Ochoa, and Samuel O. Ortiz

Mental Health Medications for Children: A Primer
Ronald T. Brown, Laura Arnstein Carpenter, and Emily Simerly

Clinical Interviews for Children and Adolescents: Assessment to Intervention
Stephanie H. McConaughy

Response to Intervention: Principles and Strategies for Effective Practice
Rachel Brown-Chidsey and Mark W. Steege

The ABCs of CBM: A Practical Guide to Curriculum-Based Measurement
Michelle K. Hosp, John L. Hosp, and Kenneth W. Howell

Fostering Independent Learning: Practical Strategies to Promote Student Success
Virginia Smith Harvey and Louise A. Chickie-Wolfe

Helping Students Overcome Substance Abuse: Effective Practices for Prevention and Intervention
Jason J. Burrow-Sanchez and Leanne S. Hawken

Helping Students Overcome Substance Abuse

Effective Practices for Prevention and Intervention

JASON J. BURROW-SANCHEZ
LEANNE S. HAWKEN

THE GUILFORD PRESS
New York   London

© 2007 The Guilford Press
A Division of Guilford Publications, Inc.
72 Spring Street, New York, NY 10012
www.guilford.com

Printed in Canada

This book is printed on acid-free paper.

Last digit is print number: 9 8 7 6 5 4 3 2 1

Library of Congress Cataloging-in-Publication Data

Burrow-Sanchez, Jason J.
  Helping students overcome substance abuse : effective practices for prevention and intervention / by Jason J. Burrow-Sanchez, Leanne S. Hawken.
    p. ; cm.—(The Guilford practical intervention in the schools series)
  Includes bibliographical references and index.
  ISBN-13: 978-1-59385-454-6 (pbk. : alk. paper)
  ISBN-10: 1-59385-454-4 (pbk. : alk. paper)
   1. School children—Substance use—United States—Prevention. 2. School mental health services—United States. I. Hawken, Leanne S. II. Title. III. Series.
   [DNLM: 1. Substance-Related Disorders—prevention & control—United States. 2. Adolescent—United States. 3. Child—United States. 4. Counseling—methods—United States. 5. Referral and Consultation—United States. 6. School Health Services—United States. WM 270 B9725h 2007]
  HV4999.C45B87 2007
  371.1′7840973—dc22

                                                                  2006036535

About the Authors

Jason J. Burrow-Sanchez, PhD, is Assistant Professor of Counseling Psychology in the Department of Educational Psychology at the University of Utah. He is a licensed psychologist, and his clinical experience includes work with adolescents struggling with substance abuse. His research interests are the prevention and treatment of substance abuse with adolescent populations in school and community settings.

Leanne S. Hawken, PhD, is Assistant Professor in the Department of Special Education at the University of Utah. Her area of research interest is positive behavior support, including schoolwide behavior support, targeted interventions for students at risk, and functional assessment/behavior support planning for students engaging in severe problem behavior.

Contents

List of Figures and Tables   xi

1. **Understanding the Context of Student Substance Use and Abuse**   1

   What Are Substance Use and Abuse?   2
   General Definitions   2
   Medically Based Terminology and Criteria   3
   Research on Student Substance Use and Abuse: National Data Sources
       and Major Use Categories   5
   Experimental Substance Use   6
   Substance Abuse   8
   Substance Dependence   9
   Substance Use and Abuse in Specific Student Populations   10
   General Student Population and School Dropouts   10
   Gender Differences   10
   Differences among Racial and Ethnic Groups   12
   Students with and without Disabilities   14
   Federal Laws and School Policies Relevant to Student Substance Abuse   16
   The Family Educational Rights and Privacy Act   16
   Title 42 of the U.S. Code of Federal Regulations, Part 2   17
   Zero Tolerance Policies   20
   Case Example   21
   Chapter Summary   23
   Chapter Resources   23

2. **Development and Maintenance of Substance Abuse**   25

   Why Do Some Students Abuse Substances?   25
   Biologically Based Theories of Substance Abuse   26
   The Disease Model   26
   Brain Chemistry   27
   Genetic Factors   28

Social Learning Theory of Substance Abuse   29
    Social Learning, Behavioral, and Cognitive-Behavioral Theories   29
    Substance Use as a Coping Skill   29
    Modeling   30
    Self-Efficacy Expectations   30
Risk and Protective Factors for Student Substance Abuse   31
    Ecology of Risk and Protective Factors   31
    Defining Risk and Protective Factors   32
    Major Categories of Risk and Protective Factors   33
Case Example   39
Chapter Summary   42
Chapter Resources   42

3. Knowing Drugs of Abuse and Screening for a Substance Abuse Problem   **44**
Major Substances of Abuse   45
    Depressants   45
    Stimulants   50
    Opioids   51
    Club Drugs   52
    Marijuana   53
    Inhalants   54
Screening for a Substance Abuse Problem   55
    Issues of Consent and Confidentiality   56
    Defining Screening and Assessment for a Substance Problem   57
    Establishing a Positive Working Relationship   58
Steps in the Screening Process   60
    Step 1: Is Screening Necessary?   60
    Step 2: Conduct a Screening   62
    Step 3: Decide on Need for Assessment   64
    Step 4: Follow-Up   65
Case Example   65
Chapter Summary   67
Chapter Resources   67

4. Prevention Programming   **69**
The Three Levels of Prevention Programming   69
Principles of Drug Abuse Prevention   71
Evaluating Research-Based Prevention Programs   73
    Evaluation of a Universal Prevention Program: LifeSkills Training   74
    Evaluation of a Selected (or Indicated) Prevention Program:
        Project Towards No Drug Abuse   75
    Evaluation of an Indicated Prevention Program: Reconnecting Youth   77
    Evaluation of a Tiered Program: Adolescent Transitions Program   79
    Summary of Research-Based Prevention Programs   81
Evaluating the Drug Abuse Resistance Education Program   81
    Evaluation Studies of D.A.R.E.   82
    Core Elements of D.A.R.E.   83
    Why Is D.A.R.E. So Popular?   84
Planning for Implementation of a Substance Abuse Prevention Program   85
    What Is the Severity of the Problem?   86
    Is the School Ready to Implement a Substance Abuse Prevention Program?   88
    What Are the Existing Gaps in Services for Students?   91
    In What Ways Can the School Collaborate with the Local Community?   91

Case Example   91
Chapter Summary   94
Chapter Resources   94

5. Individual Interventions   96
ERIN M. INGOLDSBY *and* DAVID EHRMAN
Types of Individual Interventions for Substance-Using Adolescents   97
  How Are Substance-Using Adolescents Currently Treated?   98
  Effectiveness of Current Interventions   104
Important Questions about Individual Interventions for Students   106
  What Are the Essential Components of Student Interventions?   106
  *When Should a School Mental Health Professional Decide to Implement
    an Individual Intervention Plan?*   106
  *What Is the School Professional's Role When the Student Is Receiving Treatment
    from an Outside Agency?*   107
A Comprehensive Early Intervention Program   110
  The Basis for Our Intervention Program   112
  *A Brief Adolescent-Focused, School-Based Intervention
    for Substance Use*   113
  Special Issues in Intervening with Substance-Using Students   122
Case Example   124
Chapter Summary   126
Chapter Resources   127

6. Group Interventions   130
Types of Group Interventions   130
  Psychoeducational Groups   131
  Support Groups   131
  Self-Help Groups   132
  Therapy Groups   133
Understanding the Developmental Process of Groups   133
  Initial Stage   134
  Transition Stage   136
  Working Stage   137
  Termination Stage   137
  A Note about Group Stages   138
Group Leadership Skills   138
  Basic Counseling Skills   139
  Modeling Desired Behaviors   142
  Confrontation   142
  Working with Resistant Members   143
  Cultural Awareness and Competency   145
Practical Considerations of Group Work in Schools   147
  Developing a Group Plan   147
  Group Logistics   151
  Confidentiality   154
  Member Goals   156
  Support from the Larger System   157
  Specific Issues for Substance-Abuse-Related Groups   157
Case Example   158
Chapter Summary   160
Chapter Resources   160

7. **Consultation and Referral**   163

CLAUDIA G. VINCENT

Overview of the Key Features of the Consultation and Referral Process   164
Practical Steps for Non-School-Based Service Delivery   166
   Identifying the Need for Community-Based Services   166
   Gathering Critical Pieces of Information to Shape an Action Plan   170
   Locating Available Resources   177
   Matching Available Services with a Student's Needs   179
   Putting It All Together   186
Considering Financial Responsibilities   188
Building and Maintaining a Systemic Referral Process   189
   Team-Based Approach   190
   Mutual Education   190
   Responsiveness to Existing Policies   190
Case Example   191
Chapter Summary   193
Chapter Resources   194

References   195

Index   205

List of Figures and Tables

FIGURES

FIGURE 1.1. Lifetime prevalence rates—Monitoring the Future (MTF) 2004.   7

FIGURE 1.2. Annual prevalence rates—MTF 2004.   8

FIGURE 1.3. Past-30-day prevalence rates—MTF 2004.   9

FIGURE 1.4. Lifetime prevalence rates for 12th-grade male and female students, 1996–2000.   11

FIGURE 1.5. Past-30-day prevalence rates for 12th-grade male and female students, 1996–2000.   11

FIGURE 1.6. Annual prevalence rates by racial/ethnic group for any illicit drug—MTF 2002–2003.   12

FIGURE 1.7. Past-30-day prevalence rates by racial/ethnic group for alcohol—MTF 2002–2003.   13

FIGURE 1.8. Past-30-day prevalence rates for 12th-grade females by ethnicity, 1996–2000.   14

FIGURE 1.9. Past-30-day prevalence rates for 12th-grade males by ethnicity, 1996–2000.   15

FIGURE 1.10. Sample Release of Information Form.   19

FIGURE 2.1. Ecological model of development.   32

FIGURE 3.1. Student Screening Decision Sheet (SSDS).   61

FIGURE 4.1. Prevention triangle.   70

FIGURE 4.2. School Readiness Form.   90

FIGURE 5.1. Guidelines for matching student needs with intervention settings.   108

FIGURE 5.2. Decisional Balance Worksheet.   116

FIGURE 5.3. Change Plan Worksheet.   117

FIGURE 5.4. Personal Goal Worksheet.   118

FIGURE 5.5. Functional Assessment Worksheet.   119

FIGURE 5.6. Decisional Balance Worksheet, with guidelines for the school mental   120
health professional.

FIGURE 5.7. Change Plan Worksheet, with guidelines for the school mental   121
health professional.

FIGURE 6.1. Continuum of group types for adolescent substance use and abuse.   131

FIGURE 6.2. Stages of group development.   134

FIGURE 6.3. Outline for a student aftercare group.   149

FIGURE 7.1. Coordinating treatment for students with substance abuse   187
and related problems.

FIGURE 7.2. An integrated systemic approach to consultation and referral.   191

TABLES

TABLE 2.1. Risk and Protective Factors for Adolescent Substance Use and Abuse   34

TABLE 2.2. Ray's Risk and Protective Factors for Substance Abuse   41

TABLE 3.1. Drugs of Abuse   46

TABLE 3.2. Screening Measures   64

TABLE 5.1. Suggested Structure for Intervention Based on MET and CBT   111

TABLE 7.1. Overview of Continuum of Services   181

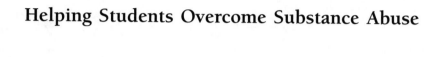

Helping Students Overcome Substance Abuse

1

Understanding the Context
of Student Substance Use and Abuse

The current national data on substance use by middle and high school students leave no question that a segment of this population is experimenting with, regularly using, or actively abusing psychoactive substances (Johnston, O'Malley, Bachman, & Schulenberg, 2005). Substance use and abuse are issues that we school mental health professionals will almost inevitably encounter in our work settings. Indeed, probably few of us do *not* know of a student who is experiencing or has experienced a problem with alcohol or other drugs. The good news is that many important advances have been made in both prevention of and intervention in adolescent substance abuse. Substance abuse by students in middle and high schools is the focus of this book. There are many good resources (e.g., scholarly books, research articles) on the topic of substance abuse; however, few of them focus on the specific needs of mental health professionals who are addressing these issues in educational settings. Therefore, we have designed this book to be a practical and user-friendly guide for such professionals who work in middle and high school settings.

Our purpose in this book is to provide school mental health professionals with up-to-date and research-based information in the areas of adolescent substance abuse prevalence, assessment, prevention, group interventions, individual interventions, and the referral process. We realize that you—the professionals reading this book—are required to practice within the contexts of your schools, and that each school follows its own set of practices, procedures, and laws regarding student substance use and abuse. You will need to consider your own school and district policies as well as applicable state and federal laws regarding student substance abuse, but you can use this book to learn effective ways to work with students who are experiencing problems with substances. If you are not familiar with these policies and laws, then now is a great time to acquaint yourself with

1

them as you read this book. We have observed that many school mental health professionals are not familiar with applicable state and federal laws regarding substance use. In addition, some personnel feel they are not in a position to have much impact when a student experiences problems with substances. For example, many schools across the nation have *zero tolerance* policies that are carried out by school administrators, who enforce negative consequences for the students involved. In most cases, this means that the students are suspended or expelled from school, depending on the circumstances. These students are not likely to receive much support from school mental health professionals in actually addressing their problems with substances. Furthermore, when a student returns to school following a drug-related suspension, the issue of substance abuse is not typically addressed by school personnel; if a student is expelled for a substance-related incident, the student's substance problem is no longer seen as an issue at that particular school.

School personnel may also argue that student substance abuse is not their responsibility, because schools should focus strictly on academics. However, a strong argument can be made that poor mental health or engaging in risky social behaviors, including substance abuse, can negatively influence students' academic success. In fact, high school dropouts are more likely to use substances than students who stay in school (Mensch & Kandel, 1988). In other words, preventing student substance use may be one way that school mental health professionals can assist in preventing school dropout.

The purpose of this first chapter is to provide readers with a foundation for better understanding student substance use and abuse. First we provide definitions for common terms used in the field of substance abuse treatment, as well as the diagnostic criteria for substance abuse and dependence as psychiatric disorders. Then use/abuse prevalence rates for different grade levels, for boys versus girls, and for different racial/ethnic groups are provided. In addition, we discuss the major federal legislation and school policies related to student substance abuse. Finally, we include a case example in order to illustrate the information presented in this chapter. At the end of this chapter (and of each chapter in this book) is a "Chapter Resources" section, which provides the reader with a listing of relevant websites and other sources of information on the chapter topic.

WHAT ARE SUBSTANCE USE AND ABUSE?

General Definitions

First we need to consider what the terms *substance use* and *substance abuse* mean and how they differ. We define *substance use* as simply a student's previous or current use of alcohol or other drugs. Many adolescents experiment with these substances or use them occasionally, but do not go on to develop substance abuse problems (Newcomb, 1995; Shelder & Block, 1990). In other words, the fact that a student is using or has used a substance does not necessarily mean that he or she is abusing that substance. In fact, some authorities argue that experimentation with drugs or engaging in other risk-taking behaviors is a "normal" part of adolescent social development (Yagamuchi & Kandel, 1984). Of course, this is only true if an adolescent does not actually develop a problem with substances as a result of using them. Unfortunately, however, some adolescents who use substances will then go on to experience problems related to their use. Thus, we define *substance abuse* as the experiencing of significant problems (e.g., school, personal, family) related to substance use. So far we have defined both of these terms somewhat generally, but the definitions will be helpful as you read through this book. (We provide a more precise medical definition of substance abuse below.)

Throughout the book, we use the terms *substance* and *drug* synonymously. Certain substances of abuse are legal and can be readily purchased, including alcohol and tobacco. Both of these substances, however, are only legal for persons meeting specific age requirements (e.g., age 21 for alcohol). Other substances of abuse are only legal when prescribed by a medical doctor. These substances include narcotics-based pain medications (e.g., OxyContin) and certain psychostimulants (e.g., Ritalin). Still other substances of abuse are generally illegal regardless of the situation, including marijuana, methamphetamine, and hallucinogens (e.g., LSD). Therefore, for the purposes of this book, the term *substances* refers to all drugs that are illegal for students in middle or high schools to possess or use.

Medically Based Terminology and Criteria

Up to this point, we have been discussing substance use and abuse fairly generally, in order to promote a better understanding of the major distinction between the two terms. However, other terms used throughout this book in relation to substance abuse need to be defined; these terms include *symptom, syndrome, disorder,* and *co-occurring.* The official diagnostic criteria for substance abuse and substance dependence also need to be set forth. Although these terms and criteria are rooted in the medical field as opposed to being educational in nature, school mental health professionals need to understand them because of their common usage among health care professionals in the field of substance abuse. Because the services for addressing student substance abuse typically involve the coordinated efforts of professionals from both educational and medical settings, it is important that school mental health professionals have some knowledge of the language commonly used by their medical colleagues.

Symptom, Syndrome, and Disorder

We begin by defining common terms used in relation to the diagnostic criteria for substance use disorders. A *symptom* of substance abuse is a behavior or emotion related to the problem, such as excessive absences from school due to drug use. A substance abuse *syndrome* comprises many symptoms related to the problem, such as excessive school absences, problems with others due to drug use (e.g., arguments with parents), and legal problems due to drugs (e.g., charges of drug possession). A set of symptoms or a syndrome is called a *disorder* when it meets the specific diagnostic criteria described in an accepted classification system.

Criteria for Substance Abuse and Dependence as Disorders

One of the most commonly used systems for classifying disorders in medical and mental health settings is the *Diagnostic and Statistical Manual of Mental Disorders*, fourth edition, text revision (DSM-IV-TR; American Psychiatric Association, 2000). It should be noted that some experts believe (see Winters, 2001) that the criteria set forth in the DSM-IV-TR are not entirely appropriate for diagnosing adolescent substance problems, for reasons that will be addressed further below and in Chapter 3. However, we provide the DSM-IV-TR criteria here because the majority of medical and other mental health professionals use them as the basis for diagnosing an adolescent with a substance-related disorder. The DSM-IV-TR includes a general category of *substance use disorders*, in which *substance abuse* and *substance dependence* are defined by specific criteria. The diagnostic criteria for substance abuse disorder include one (or more) of the following symptoms within the past 12 months: (1) failure to fulfill major role obligations (e.g., excessive absences from school) due to recurring substance use; (2) recurring substance use in hazardous situations (e.g., driving under the influence); (3) recurring legal problems related to substance use (e.g., citation for possessing an illegal drug); or (4) continued use of substances despite persisting interpersonal problems (e.g., arguments with parents).

The diagnostic criteria for substance dependence disorder include three (or more) of the following in the same 12-month period: (1) symptoms of drug tolerance (e.g., needing more of a drug to get high, or failure of the same amount of the drug to produce a substantial high); (2) symptoms of withdrawal (e.g., physical, mental, or other problems related to not using the drug, or use of the drug to avoid such problems); (3) taking the drug in greater amounts or over a longer period of time than originally intended; (4) a constant need for, or unsuccessful efforts to reduce or stop, the drug use; (5) spending a lot of time in activities related to either obtaining the drug, using the drug, or recovering from the physiological or mental effects of the drug (e.g., hangovers); (6) either giving up or limiting participation in activities (e.g., school, work, social) that had importance prior to the use of drugs; or (7) continuing to use the drug in spite of awareness that such use may have caused or worsened other physical or psychological problems (e.g., using alcohol despite knowing that it exacerbates a preexisting problem with depression).

Tolerance and Withdrawal

Two important terms in the DSM-IV-TR definition of substance dependence disorder are *tolerance* and *withdrawal*, both of which are often misunderstood. *Tolerance* is generally defined as the need for more of a substance to obtain the same desired effect (American Psychiatric Association, 2000). For example, coffee drinkers may start out only needing small amounts of the substance (e.g., 1/2 to 1 full cup) to experience the stimulating effects of caffeine. Over time, however, they usually develop a tolerance to caffeine and frequently report needing more of the substance (e.g., 2–3 cups) to experience the same desired effects from caffeine.

Withdrawal is generally defined as the experience of unpleasant physical or psychological symptoms related to reducing or stopping the use of a drug (American Psychiatric Association, 2000). To take the example above a step further, coffee drinkers frequently report experiencing such symptoms as irritability, slowness, or headaches when they do not get their "daily dose" of coffee. These unpleasant symptoms are typically relieved after drinking a cup of coffee (or more!). It should be noted that all drugs do not produce the same intensity of tolerance and withdrawal symptoms. Certain drugs (e.g., barbiturates) are more likely to produce noticeable symptoms of tolerance and withdrawal, whereas for other drugs (e.g., marijuana) the symptoms will be more subtle, and DSM-IV-TR defines formal withdrawal symptoms only for drugs in the first group. Generally speaking, symptoms of tolerance and withdrawal are produced by the body's gradual physical and psychological adaptation to the frequent use of a substance.

Co-Occurrence of Substance Use and Other Disorders

The findings from current research suggest that a substantial number of youth with a substance use disorder are simultaneously experiencing another disorder. For example, Riggs (2003) reports the following co-occurring disorders and their prevalence for adolescents with a substance use disorder: conduct disorders (60–80%); attention-deficit/hyperactivity disorder or ADHD (30–50%); depressive disorders (15–25%); anxiety disorders (15–25%); and bipolar disorder (10–15%). A frequently asked question regarding co-occurring disorders is "Which disorder came first?" For example, did an adolescent experiencing depression begin using a drug (e.g., methamphetamine) to alleviate the depression? Or did an adolescent with a drug problem develop depression due to experiencing the "lows" of withdrawal from methamphetamine? These are not easy questions for which absolute answers can be provided. In work with a student who is experiencing a problem with substances along with another disorder, it is best to determine the history of each problem. For example, which disorder was present initially, and how did the other disorder develop in relation to the initial disorder? Research on the developmental pathways of adolescent substance abuse suggests that many youth with substance abuse problems experienced other disorders (e.g., mental, learning) earlier in their lives (Tarter, 2002). This suggests that a student experiencing a mental health disorder such as depression or anxiety is at higher risk for developing a substance use disorder, especially if the initial disorder is not treated appropriately.

RESEARCH ON STUDENT SUBSTANCE USE AND ABUSE: NATIONAL DATA SOURCES AND MAJOR USE CATEGORIES

Among the questions we are commonly asked are "How much are adolescents using drugs in the United States? And what types of drugs are they using?" The federal government spends substantial amounts of money annually to fund research programs to answer these very questions. Many different research programs coordinated by many government agencies (e.g., the National Institutes of Health, the Centers for Disease Control and Prevention), as well as by several universities, examine the substance use behaviors of children, adolescents, and adults in the United States. We mainly concern ourselves in this section with the findings from two major ongoing research programs that examine the prevalence rates of such behaviors among students and youth. We describe these research programs here because we refer to their data throughout this book.

One major source of information is the Monitoring the Future (MTF) studies, which are conducted annually by the University of Michigan's Institute for Social Research and funded by the National Institute on Drug Abuse (NIDA). From 1975 through 1990, the MTF researchers collected data on 12th-grade students' drug use; beginning in 1991, students from grades 8 and 10 were added to expand the sample range. Substance use rates are obtained annually from a nationally representative sample of approximately 45,000 students in grades 8, 10, and 12 from 400 schools. Data are collected for the MTF studies by asking students to complete a series of questions on substance use and related topics during a class period. The results from these studies are made available to the public on the MTF website (*www.monitoringthefuture.org*).

A second major source of substance use prevalence data is the National Survey on Drug Use and Health (NSDUH). The NSDUH began in 1971, and researchers collect data from a nationally representative sample of civilians, excluding institutionalized individuals (e.g., prisoners). Since 1991, the survey has been conducted annually and is funded by the U.S. government's Substance Abuse and Mental Health Services Administration (SAMHSA). Approximately 70,000 individuals ages 12 and older are interviewed each year about drug use and other health-related behaviors. In particular, data are collected from youth ages 12–17 about their drug use behaviors. In contrast to the MTF studies, the NSDUH research includes samples of youth who have dropped out of school. The NSDUH results are available to the public at one of SAMHSA's websites (*www.oas.samhsa.gov*).

We have discussed above how the DSM-IV-TR separates substance use disorders into two categories: substance abuse and substance dependence. This classification scheme is based largely on research with adults and requires special consideration when applied to children and adolescents. In fact, Winters (2001) recommends that adolescent substance use be considered along a continuum of severity from no or little use at one end to severe use at the other end. This conceptualization implies that adolescent substance use (and related problems) is graduated over time rather than being an all-or-nothing event. In order to make the most sense of the data provided by national studies, we consider the prevalence of substance use in terms of three major categories: *experimental substance use*, substance *abuse*, and substance *dependence*.

Experimental Substance Use

We define the *experimental use* of a substance as a student's trying a particular substance (such as alcohol) once or very infrequently, but not going far beyond that level. Such a student may say, "I've tried beer once at a party and didn't like it," or "Occasionally I'll have a beer at a party, but not very often." As mentioned above, some researchers suggest that experimentation with substances and other risky behaviors are typical aspects of adolescent development (Yagamuchi & Kandel, 1984). Adolescents with parents who have strict standards against drug use may be uncomfortable sharing their experimental use history, for fear that their parents will not believe that they have only used a substance once or very infrequently. Self-reports of experimental drug use by adolescents should also be tempered with the knowledge that some adolescents will report *lower* levels than they actually use, especially when they are first questioned about their drug use history (Stinchfield, 1997).

Much of the information we have about experimental substance use by students at the national level comes from the MTF studies described above. In these studies, students are asked to report their use of substances in their lifetimes; for example, the question "Have you ever used alcohol in your lifetime?" is used to ascertain whether a student has ever used alcohol. The responses to these types of questions provide estimates of experimental use rates for students at the secondary level.

The lifetime prevalence rates obtained from a recent MTF study for secondary students across a number of substances are presented in Figure 1.1 (Johnston et al., 2005). As can be seen from this figure, alcohol, cigarettes, and marijuana are the three most commonly reported substances used by students in grades 8, 10, and 12 during their lifetimes. After these three substances, sharp declines in experimental use are indicated for drugs such as methamphetamine, hallucinogens, and tranquilizers.

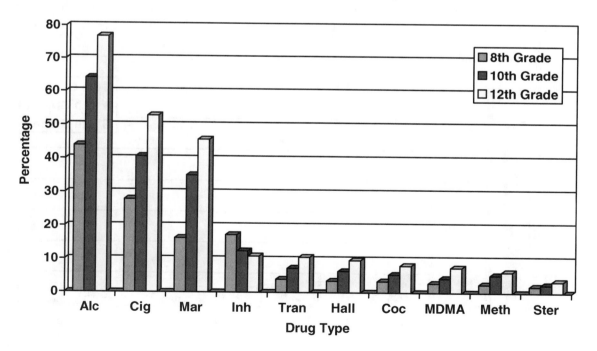

FIGURE 1.1. Lifetime prevalence rates—Monitoring the Future (MTF) 2004. Data from Johnston, O'Malley, Bachman, and Schulenberg (2005). Alc, alcohol; Cig, cigarettes; Mar, marijuana; Inh, inhalants; Tran, tranquilizers; Hall, hallucinogens; Coc, cocaine; MDMA, Ecstasy; Meth, methamphetamine; Ster, steroids.

Of all the substances listed in Figure 1.1, alcohol is the one students experiment with the most. This finding is probably not surprising, given that alcohol is a highly accessible substance in the United States and can usually be obtained with little difficulty (albeit illegally) even by minors. Students are also exposed to many media images of adults consuming alcoholic beverages, such as television commercials, billboards, and magazine advertisements. In addition, adolescents who observe substance use by parents or older siblings are at elevated risk for trying substances themselves (Hawkins, Catalano, & Miller, 1992).

Substance Abuse

As described above, the DSM-IV-TR diagnostic criteria indicate that the use of substances progresses to *substance abuse* when an individual has experienced certain drug-related problems within the past 12 months. For students, such problems can take the form of declines in academic performance, excessive absences, reckless driving, frequently arguing with adults about their drug use, or problems with the legal system. In order to get an idea of substance abuse prevalence rates in the secondary student population, we have defined these rates in terms of the reported use of drugs by students within the past year.

As part of the MTF studies, students are asked to report their levels of substance use for the past year. Again, based on the DSM diagnostic criteria, we consider these rates to be rough indicators of the number of students whose substance use has progressed to substance abuse. As can be seen in Figure 1.2 for a recent MTF study (Johnston et al., 2005), the rates of substance use for students in the past year drop below the lifetime use

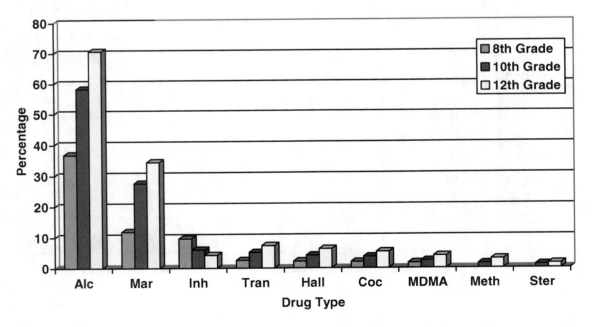

FIGURE 1.2. Annual prevalence rates—MTF 2004. Data from Johnston et al. (2005). Abbreviations as in Figure 1.1.

rates presented in Figure 1.1, but alcohol and marijuana (data on annual rates of cigarette use were not available in this study) remain two of the most commonly reported substances used.

Substance Dependence

As also described above, substance abuse progresses to *substance dependence* when a student experiences physical and psychological symptoms related to problems with controlling the use of a substance, as outlined in the DSM-IV-TR criteria. These physical and psychological symptoms can take the form of needing more of the substance to obtain the same effect (i.e., tolerance), experiencing unpleasantness when the substance is not used (i.e., withdrawal), persistent but unsuccessful efforts to control use, or giving up previously enjoyable activities (e.g., playing soccer) in favor of using substances. Based on the DSM-IV-TR criteria, we consider student-reported rates of substance use within the past 30 days to be rough indicators of the number of students who have progressed from substance abuse to substance dependence. The past-30-days data from a recent MTF study (Johnston et al., 2005) can be seen in Figure 1.3. Similar to the data presented above, alcohol, cigarettes, and marijuana are the substances reported by secondary students to be the most commonly used during this time period.

Generally speaking, substance dependence is characterized by an individual's experiencing a loss of control over the substance and saying things such as "I can't control my

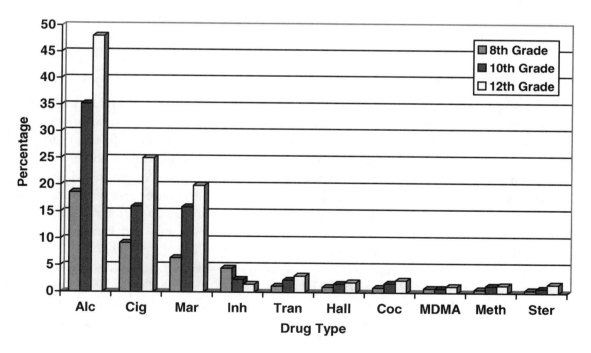

FIGURE 1.3. Past-30-day prevalence rates—MTF 2004. Data from Johnston et al. (2005). Abbreviations as in Figure 1.1.

use no matter how hard I try," or "I've tried many times to quit, but it never works." These types of symptoms are more likely to be seen in older adolescents and adults who have been using substances over a considerable amount of time. In addition, certain drugs such as cocaine and methamphetamine are highly physiologically addictive, which can act to expedite the transition from experimental use to substance dependence.

SUBSTANCE USE AND ABUSE IN SPECIFIC STUDENT POPULATIONS

General Student Population and School Dropouts

As described above, substance use is prevalent among the general student population at the secondary level. Consistent trends over time indicate that substance use gradually increases from 8th to 12th grade. The substances used most frequently by students across grade levels are alcohol, cigarettes, and marijuana; beyond these three substances, the use rates for other substances decrease, with slight variations across demographic subgroups (e.g., gender, race/ethnicity). In this section we discuss the differences in rates between genders and among racial/ethnic groups, but first a word about one consequence of our reliance on *student* data is in order: Typically, school-based prevalence studies do not account for the drug use rates of school dropouts. In fact, as noted earlier, high school dropouts are likely than students who stay in school to report higher drug use rates (Mensch & Kandel, 1988). Thus students who drop out of school are a high-risk group for substance abuse, but are not accounted for in the national school-based prevalence studies on substance use.

Gender Differences

A common perception is that male students use or abuse substances at higher rates than female students. In general, this perception is accurate, but the actual disparity between male and female substance use is not as large as commonly believed. To illustrate this point, data are presented in Figure 1.4 from a study conducted by Wallace and colleagues (2003). The data from this study were a subsample of the data collected in the MTF studies. As can be seen from Figure 1.4, male students in the 12th grade reported higher levels of use than female students for all substances listed, with the exception of stimulants. Note, however, that the difference between the use rates of male and female students across drug categories is relatively small.

Figure 1.5 displays the reported levels of substance use in the past 30 days by male and female students in the 12th grade (Wallace et al., 2003). These data indicate that male students reported higher use rates than female students with respect to each substance (stimulants are very close), but again the differences are not marked. The data from Figures 1.4 and 1.5 thus suggest that while in general male students report higher substance use rates, female students should not be overlooked with respect to substance abuse concerns.

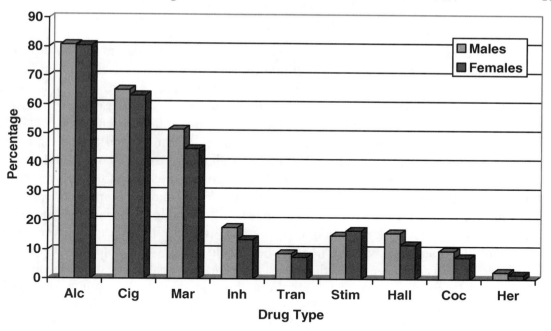

FIGURE 1.4. Lifetime prevalence rates for 12th-grade male and female students, 1996–2000. Data from Wallace et al. (2003). Stim, stimulants; Her, heroin; other abbreviations as in Figure 1.1.

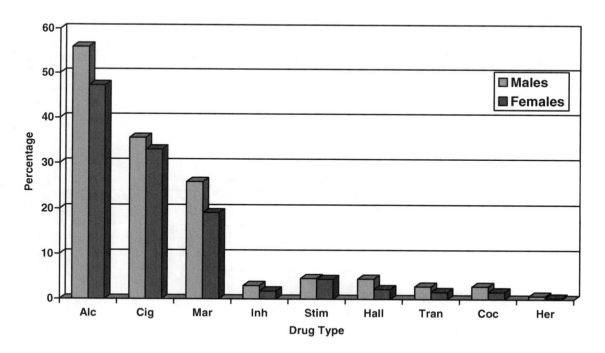

FIGURE 1.5. Past-30-day prevalence rates for 12th-grade male and female students, 1996–2000. Data from Wallace et al. (2003). Abbreviations as in Figures 1.1 and 1.4.

Differences among Racial and Ethnic Groups

Data collected as part of the MTF studies provide us with information on the drug use rates among the three largest racial and ethnic student groups—that is, European American, Hispanic, and African American (Johnston, O'Malley, Bachman, & Schulenberg, 2004). The annual prevalence rates for use of any illicit drug among these three groups of students across three grade levels are displayed in Figure 1.6 (Johnston et al., 2004). In this study, *illicit drugs* were defined as any substances that are illegal to use for recreational purposes; in other words, this class includes all drugs except alcohol and tobacco. As can be seen from Figure 1.6, Hispanic students reported the highest use rates in grade 8 but fell behind European American students in grades 10 and 12. Some of this dropoff in substance use rates for Hispanic students may be attributable to the fact that these students are at the highest risk for school dropout, and therefore these prevalence rates do not account for adolescents who are not in school (Shin, 2005). Also, note from Figure 1.6 that African American students had the lowest use rates across all three grade levels. This overall trend in substance use rates for these three student groups holds for certain drugs. As can be seen from Figure 1.7, the past-30-day rates of use for alcohol (Johnston et al., 2004) are similar to the annual illicit drug use rates presented in Figure 1.6 for each student group. However, certain drugs (not illustrated) have higher use rates within specific racial and ethnic groups. For example, Hispanic students reported higher levels of use for crack and heroin than did European Americans and African Americans (Johnston et al., 2004).

So far we have only considered the differences among substance use rates for students from the three largest, most broadly defined racial and ethnic minority groups: European American, African American, and Hispanic. What about the substance use

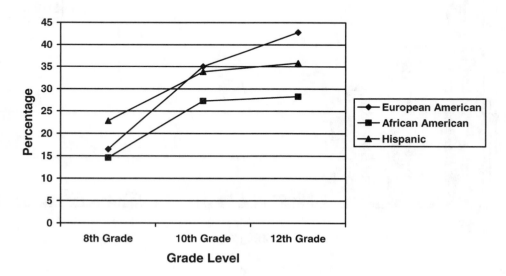

FIGURE 1.6. Annual prevalence rates by racial/ethnic group for any illicit drug—MTF 2002–2003. Data from Johnston, O'Malley, Bachman, and Schulenberg (2004).

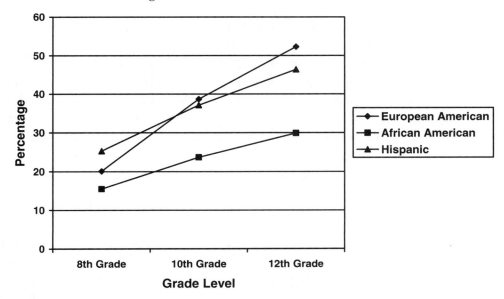

FIGURE 1.7. Past-30-day prevalence rates by racial/ethnic group for alcohol—MTF 2002–2003. Data from Johnston et al. (2004).

rates for students from other racial and ethnic minority groups in the United States, as well as for particular subgroups of Hispanic students? Wallace and his colleagues (2003) compared the substance use levels among various racial and ethnic minority groups of students by averaging their use rates across a 5-year period (1996–2000), so that each group would have an adequate sample size for comparison purposes. Figure 1.8 contains the past-30-day substance use rates for female students in the 12th grade across racial and ethnic groups over this 5-year period. As can be seen from this figure, American Indian female students reported higher substance use rates for alcohol, cigarettes, marijuana, inhalants, and stimulants than did female students from other groups. Figure 1.8 also indicates several subgroup differences for Hispanic students. (The term *Hispanic* includes people whose origins are in many geographic regions, including Mexico, Puerto Rico, Cuba, and various Central and South American countries.) For instance, Mexican American female students reported higher levels of alcohol use than Puerto Rican female students, whereas the reverse was true for marijuana.

Now let us consider the substance use rates for male students across these same racial and ethnic groups. Figure 1.9 depicts the average substance use rates for male students in the 12th grade from these groups over the same 5-year period (Wallace et al., 2003). The figure indicates that European American and Mexican American students reported the first and second highest rates of alcohol use, respectively, and that these were the highest rates for any drug listed. For cigarettes, male American Indian students reported the highest use rates, followed by European American students. For marijuana, male Mexican American students reported the highest use rates, followed by American Indian students and students from the other Hispanic subgroups listed. It is clear from these data that considerable variation in substance use exists among male students from different racial and ethnic groups.

We now briefly compare substance use rates for the female and male students presented in Figures 1.8 and 1.9, respectively. For alcohol, male students from each racial and ethnic group reported higher levels of use than their female counterparts did. For cigarettes, marijuana, and stimulants, American Indian female students reported the highest levels of use across any of the groups listed, regardless of gender.

Students with and without Disabilities

The findings from available research suggest that students with disabilities are at high risk for the use and abuse of substances (Fowler & Tisdale, 1992; Karacostas & Fisher, 1993; Maag, Irvin, Reid, & Vasa, 1994). However, large-scale studies on substance use and abuse for these students are lacking; thus we are not able to provide detailed prevalence rates like those provided above for students in general education. In general, the limited research available suggests that students with disabilities are at higher risk for substance abuse than students in general education classes. For example, two studies found that students with learning disabilities were at higher risk for substance use and abuse than were students without learning disabilities (Karacostas & Fisher, 1993; Maag et al., 1994).

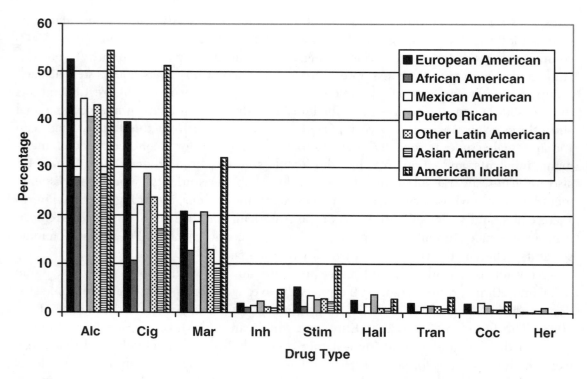

FIGURE 1.8. Past-30-day prevalence rates for 12th-grade females by ethnicity, 1996–2000. Data from Wallace et al. (2003). Abbreviations as in Figures 1.1 and 1.4.

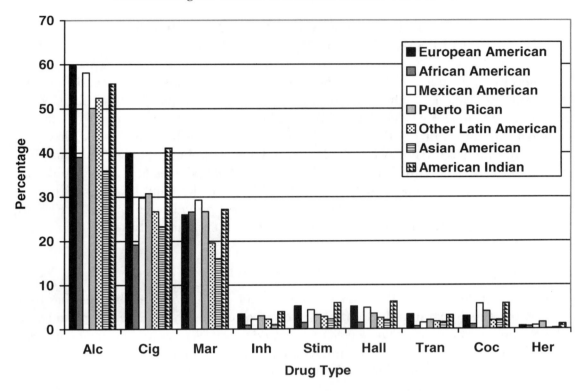

FIGURE 1.9. Past-30-day prevalence rates for 12th-grade males by ethnicity, 1996–2000. Data from Wallace et al. (2003). Abbreviations as in Figures 1.1 and 1.4.

Some researchers suggest that disability-specific factors place students at higher risk for substance abuse (McCombs & Moore, 2002). For example, a student with a learning disability may experience impaired decision making and thus be more susceptible to peer pressure to use substances. A student with an emotional disturbance may be more likely to experience a stressful home environment or to have a parent who uses substances. A student with a developmental disability may have impaired ability to make judgments about the risks associated with using a substance. As described above, many students with substance use disorders also experience co-occurring learning disabilities or ADHD (Riggs, 2003; Tarter, 2002). In addition, because students with disabilities are often prescribed psychotropic medications to manage one or more co-occurring disorders, these students are at risk for combining prescribed medication with alcohol and illicit drugs.

In schools, much of the prevention programming for substance abuse is targeted toward students in general education classes (Fowler & Tisdale, 1992; McCombs & Moore, 2002). This suggests that the needs of students with disabilities are not generally taken into account when preventive interventions are developed and implemented within schools. It is our hope that more research will be conducted in this area, so that we may better understand the specific needs of these students in relation to substance abuse.

FEDERAL LAWS AND SCHOOL POLICIES
RELEVANT TO STUDENT SUBSTANCE ABUSE

Two pieces of federal legislation that are relevant to student substance use and abuse are the Family Educational Rights and Privacy Act (FERPA) and Title 42 of the U.S. Code of Federal Regulations, Part 2 (42 CFR). We have found that most school mental health professionals are aware of FERPA and its basic tenets, but we have also found that most school professionals are not aware of 42 CFR and how it applies to student substance use and abuse. In addition, there are federally related school policies for student substance abuse commonly known as *zero tolerance*, of which school mental health professionals have varying amounts of knowledge. Therefore, we next provide an overview of FERPA, 42 CFR, and zero tolerance policies related to student substance abuse.

The Family Educational Rights and Privacy Act

FERPA, also referred to as the Buckley Amendment, was enacted in 1974 and has been revised since its initial introduction. The interested reader can find the complete text of FERPA online (*www.ed.gov/policy/gen/reg/ferpa/index.html*). As its full name suggests, this federal legislation is in place to protect the privacy of student educational records. An *educational record* as defined by FERPA includes records about a particular student that are kept in a file maintained by the school. These regulations apply to all schools that receive federal funding from the U.S. Department of Education at the elementary, secondary, or postsecondary level. When a student is below the age of 18, FERPA provides parents with the right to inspect their son's or daughter's educational records. When a student is age 18 (or older) or is attending a postsecondary institution (e.g., college or university), he or she is considered an *eligible student* and can request examination of his or her educational records without parental consent. Parents or eligible students also have the right to request that a school amend educational records if they believe that these are not accurate.

FERPA dictates that school personnel cannot ordinarily release a student's educational records without written consent from parents (or the student, if he or she is eligible). They can release these records under certain exceptions, including but not limited to school transfer, school audit, court order, and in case of an emergency related to health or safety. Also, school personnel are allowed to disclose information about the student to other personnel in the school without parental consent; however, such disclosures should only be made to those personnel who have a *legitimate educational interest* in the student. For example, does a teacher have a legitimate need to know that a student in one of his or her courses is attending an outpatient counseling group for substance abuse in the community? In this situation, the answer is probably no. But let us say a staff member at the outpatient treatment program wants regular academic progress reports from teachers in the classes where the student is struggling, to use as part of the student's treatment plan. In this situation, the decision to disclose is more clearly indicated, as a teacher will be providing information related to the legitimate educational interest of the student.

Now let us consider a set of federal regulations that specifically address the issue of substance-abuse-related information.

Title 42 of the U.S. Code of Federal Regulations, Part 2

42 CFR is a set of federal regulations specifically addressing confidentiality in regard to substance-abuse-related information. Whereas most school mental health professionals are aware of FERPA, we have found that many are not aware of 42 CFR or of how it pertains to the confidentiality of student substance abuse records. The specific regulations use the term *patient*; however, we have substituted the word *student*, as the regulations apply to *any individual*. These regulations were originally introduced in 1975 and have been subsequently amended. The interested reader can find the full text of 42 CFR online (*www.lac.org/pubs/gratis.html*).

42 CFR is applicable to all programs that provide "alcohol or drug abuse diagnosis, treatment or referral for treatment" (§ 2.11). Some of our readers may be thinking, "This means that 42 CFR does not apply to me, because I work in a school setting and my school does not provide diagnosis or treatment for substance abuse." Before deciding on the applicability of these regulations to your school, please read further. In addition, these regulations are applicable to any program that receives funds from "any department or agency of the United States" (§ 2.12), and such federal funding does not have to "directly pay for the alcohol or drug abuse diagnosis, treatment, or referral activities" (§ 2.12). In other words, if your school receives federal funds (most schools do), and if you or other school mental health professionals provide students with referrals for substance abuse treatment, then your school is obligated to abide by 42 CFR.

The following example should clarify the applicability of 42 CFR for school mental health professionals. Imagine that a school receives federal funding for a student academic program (e.g., reading or math) that has nothing to do with substance abuse diagnosis, treatment, or referral. However, the counselor at this school regularly provides community referrals to students and their parents for addressing substance abuse problems. This counselor would be required to follow the guidelines of 42 CFR, because (1) the school receives *federal funding*, and (2) the school counselor provides *referrals* for substance abuse treatment.

The next question our readers may be asking is "What does 42 CFR mean to me and my work with students who have substance abuse?" First, it is important to realize that 42 CFR supersedes all less restrictive local and state laws related to substance abuse records. Second, the purpose of these regulations is to guarantee confidentiality to an individual seeking substance abuse services. Given the social stigma attached to substance abuse in the United States, it makes sense that people are less likely to obtain needed services when they feel that the privacy of such services is not guaranteed. Third, under 42 CFR, school mental health professionals are prohibited from disclosing any information related to the "identity, diagnosis, prognosis, or treatment" (§ 290DD-3, 290EE-3) of any student regarding any program or activity concerning "alcoholism or alcohol abuse education, training, treatment, rehabilitation, or research" (§ 290DD-3).

These regulations also apply to drugs other than alcohol (§ 290EE-3). In practical terms, this means that neither the identity of a student receiving substance abuse services, nor anything about the type of services the student receives, may be disclosed.

The regulations of 42 CFR define *information* as any information, regardless of whether it is oral or written. For example, suppose you are a school psychologist, and a student named Joe with whom you are working was recently caught with alcohol at school and is subsequently attending a drug education class in the community as a result. The only reason you know that Joe is attending a drug education course is because he disclosed it to you during one of your meetings with him. A week after Joe disclosed this information, a school counselor who does not know Joe or his situation informs you that he or she is starting a counseling group for students who are exhibiting risky behaviors such as substance use. The school counselor asks you whether you can refer any students who would benefit from participating in such a group, and you immediately think of referring Joe. You can refer Joe to the group; however, you cannot disclose that Joe is already attending a drug education course to the school counselor unless certain conditions exist. We will now turn to a discussion of the specific exceptions to confidentiality that are allowed under 42 CFR.

Similar to other regulations governing confidentiality, 42 CFR allows disclosure of substance-abuse-related confidential information under specific conditions. One exception can occur when a student and his or her parents provide written consent for the disclosure of information to a third party (e.g., a community substance abuse treatment agency). In fact, 42 CFR provides guidelines for the minimum required elements needed for a written authorization form to disclose substance-abuse-related information (see Figure 1.10). It is also important to realize that some states allow minors (the age of a minor is defined by each state) to obtain substance abuse treatment and other types of treatment without the consent of their parents, while other states do not. You should check the laws of your state to determine whether minors at any age can obtain substance abuse treatment without parental consent. For example, under 42 CFR a minor who resides in a state that does not require parental consent for substance abuse treatment can provide his or her own written consent for disclosure of substance-abuse-related information. In contrast, consent for disclosure must be obtained by *both* the minor and parents in a state that does require parental consent for such treatment. In either case, most experts in this area would agree that involving a student's parents in his or her treatment is generally preferred unless it is contraindicated for some reason.

Another exception to 42 CFR is that disclosure of substance-abuse-related information can take place between personnel working in the same school, agency, or organization when such personnel have "a need for the information in connection with their duties that arise out of the provision of diagnosis, treatment, or referral for treatment of alcohol or drug abuse" (§ 2.12). This exception is a bit trickier, because you can probably think of instances in which a fellow staff member in your school does or does not have a legitimate need to know such information about a student. As discussed earlier, there are times when multiple personnel need to have information to best serve a particular student. As an example, if a student is attending an outpatient substance abuse group in the

Authorization for Release of Confidential Information

Date: _____

I, _____ , authorize _____

   (Name of student)   (Name of school personnel, and name of school)

to disclose confidential information to _____

                                           (Name of personnel at agency, and name of agency)

for the purposes of _____ .

                       (General reason for disclosure—e.g., coordinating substance abuse treatment, etc.)

I only authorize that these specific type(s) of information to be disclosed: _____

_____

(Describe the specific type(s) of information to be disclosed—e.g., assessment results, treatment progress information, etc.)

This authorization can be revoked by me or by my parents (if applicable) at any time. This authorization for release of information expires 90 days from the date on this form unless it is renewed in writing by all applicable parties.

_____   _____

Student's signature   Date

_____   _____

Parent's signature   Date

_____   _____

Parent's signature   Date

_____   _____

Authorized school representative's signature   Date

FIGURE 1.10. Sample Release of Information Form. (This form should be modified to fit the specific requirements of your setting.)

community, do his or her teachers need to be informed? One could argue that since the treatment takes place outside the school, the teachers do not need to know about the student's treatment services. However, what if the treatment program wants the school to provide regular updates on the student's academic progress in his or her courses? Regardless of the specific situation, it is always best practice to obtain written consent from the student and his or her parents prior to discussing treatment services in or outside of the school setting, and prior to disclosing substance-abuse-related information about the student.

A third exception to 42 CFR can occur when a school has a relationship with another agency to provide specific substance-abuse-related services for students. The other agency is referred to in 42 CFR as a *qualified service organization*. For example, some schools require drug testing of students who participate in the schools' athletic programs. Drug testing in schools commonly takes the form of urinalysis. The actual analysis, however, is usually done by an outside agency that contracts with the school to provide this service. In this example, the appropriate school personnel and the personnel from the testing agency can communicate about students' drug-testing results, given the prior contractual relationship.

In addition to the exceptions to confidentiality described above, other general exceptions include medical emergencies, reporting of suspected child abuse, crimes on school premises or against school personnel, qualified research, and audit/evaluation activities. We strongly recommend consulting 42 CFR itself (see the URL given above) for a full understanding of how these regulations regarding confidentiality (and exceptions to confidentiality) apply to specific situations in your school setting.

Zero Tolerance Policies

Most U.S. secondary schools have *zero tolerance* policies for student behavior related to guns, violence, and drugs. These have their origins in the policies the United States adopted in the 1980s to fight the "war on drugs." In particular, these policies were used to administer stiff consequences to individuals who were caught engaging in drug-related offenses (e.g., drug trafficking, drug selling), no matter how the offenses differed. For example, a person selling drugs would suffer the same consequences as someone importing drugs from a South American country. By the late 1980s and early 1990s, school districts in a few states began to adopt similar policies to punish student behaviors such as bringing weapons to school, violence, drug use, and other disruptive behaviors (Skiba, 2000). In 1994, the Gun-Free Schools Act (GFSA) was signed into law and mandated student expulsion for the possession of a firearm. Currently, in most schools zero tolerance policies include punishment based on the GFSA mandates, as well as punishment for various behaviors that are deemed objectionable but are not covered under GFSA (e.g., substance abuse). In other words, most schools provide strict punishment (usually immediate suspension or expulsion) to students for a range of unacceptable behaviors, and not all of this punishment is mandated by the federal government. Moreover, researchers have consistently found that traditional zero tolerance policies are generally not effective mechanisms for reducing student substance use or for making schools safer (Skiba, 2000). In essence, strict zero tolerance policies punish students instead of teaching them ways to make better decisions about the behavior(s) that have gotten them into trouble.

In many cases, zero tolerance policies make it difficult for school mental health professionals to provide any type of support services to a student with a substance abuse problem. In addition to the fact that students who violate school drug rules are often routinely suspended or expelled, the consequences of violating a school's zero tolerance policies are typically handled by an administrator. Some schools, however, may have an *early response* system in place that provides graduated punishment, so that the level of the substance-related offense matches the consequences received (Skiba, 2000). With an early response system, school mental health professionals are more likely to feel that they have opportunities to provide support to students with substance abuse problems rather than just punishing them. In general, we suggest that schools adopt policies that will actually allow school mental health professionals to help students deal with substance abuse. Making these types of modifications to existing zero tolerance policies in most schools would require collaboration between school mental health professionals and administrators, with the common goal of better serving the needs of students who exhibit substance abuse problems.

CASE EXAMPLE

Throughout the book, case examples like the one below are used to illustrate the key concepts discussed in each chapter. We hope that you will find these case examples helpful in understanding the material. We also encourage you to compare your own experiences with students in educational settings to these examples, in order to make them more "real" for you.

Martin was a 28-year-old male who, after finishing a graduate program in school counseling, began working at Central High School in a low-income area of the large city in which he lived. Martin's own experiences in high school had been quite different from those many of his current students were having. For example, he had attended high school in an upper-middle-class area of the same city and had gone on to college immediately after graduation. Although he knew that alcohol and drugs were available in his high school, he only drank alcohol when at parties and in limited amounts (e.g., one or two beers). In general, his social group in high school used other drugs infrequently, which influenced his drug use. When he began his position at Central High School, the other counselors told him that "drugs were a real problem" at the school; however, the school had very few resources available for students with substance abuse problems. The school administration did implement a zero tolerance policy for drugs on campus. This meant that any students caught using drugs or storing them (e.g., in lockers) on campus were referred to the school administration for disciplinary consequences, which typically consisted of suspension or expulsion. Martin learned that in the year before his arrival, almost 40 students had been suspended or expelled for issues related to drugs.

During the first trimester of his job as a school counselor, Martin observed a number of students who suffered the consequences of the zero tolerance policy related to the drug use. He also observed that many other students seemed to be experiencing problems related to drugs: He suspected that some students were suffering academically because of drug use, and he noticed that some students came from homes in which their parents or older siblings used drugs.

Martin had taken one course in graduate school on the topic of substance abuse. However, he did not feel competent to begin addressing this issue in his school without acquiring more information. He researched the topic on the Internet and found many excellent sites with information about student substance use. For example, he located national and local statistics on the substance use rates of high school students. He also learned that alcohol, cigarettes, and marijuana were the three most commonly used substances by adolescents. In addition, he found resources on the different types of drugs (e.g., methamphetamine, hallucinogens) that adolescents reported using, as well as their common street names. Finally, he found resources in his community to which he could refer parents who had concerns about their children's substance use.

Martin was eager to disseminate all this information, with the hope of reducing the problem at his school. In fact, he developed a substance abuse prevention curriculum unit that he delivered in ninth-grade health courses the following year. The unit covered facts about drugs, as well as risk and protective factors for use and abuse. He thought that students would make better choices if they actually learned some information about drug use and abuse. He was amazed at how many students (and school personnel!) had misperceptions and misinformation about drug abuse. He found that one common misperception among students was that marijuana was a "safe drug." That is, many of his students believed that marijuana did not have addictive properties and was relatively harmless to use. He always enjoyed seeing the surprised looks on students' faces when he explained that the smoke from marijuana contains more carcinogens than regular cigarette smoke. He also discussed the potential consequences of marijuana use (as determined by research), which include impaired memory, concentration, and learning, as well as frequent coughing, respiratory infections, and feelings of anxiety. In general, he found that most students seemed to appreciate the information he presented. In fact, some students told him that the information they learned in his unit had made them concerned about some of their friends' abusing substances. Part of Martin's unit included ways that peers could help peers (e.g., through referral to a school mental health professional) if they suspected substance abuse.

Due to the positive feedback that Martin received for the substance abuse prevention unit from students and teachers, it was expanded to include 10th-grade students the following year. He observed that the number of disciplinary consequences related to substance use decreased slightly during the first 2 years the curriculum was implemented. Martin felt good about the prevention curriculum unit he had developed and was encouraged by positive student and teacher reactions to it. He realized, however, that the unit needed to be updated and revised in order to stay "fresh" for the students who received it. Based on the success of his unit, he also began to engage his school's administrators in conversations about ways to make the zero tolerance policy more graduated, depending on the actual drug-related offenses. He hoped that in time the policy would be modified so that school mental health professionals could provide assistance to students who experienced drug problems, rather than just suspending them.

CHAPTER SUMMARY

The primary goal of this chapter is to introduce the topic of student substance abuse to school mental health professionals. In part, this has been accomplished by discussing the terminology used in the field of substance abuse treatment, with which school professionals should be familiar. We have provided general definitions of terms such as *substance use* and *substance abuse*, as well as the substance use disorder classifications presented in the DSM-IV-TR. Information on the prevalence of co-occurring mental health disorders such as ADHD, depression, and anxiety has been presented as well. Furthermore, current national prevalence rates for substance use have been presented for certain time periods (lifetime, past year, past 30 days) and for specific groups (males vs. females, racial/ethnic groupings), in order to provide school professionals with an accurate picture of adolescent use rates. Federal legislation (FERPA and 42 CFR) and zero tolerance policies have then been discussed, because school professionals need to be aware of how these regulations and policies apply to student substance use and abuse issues in their schools. Finally, a case example has illustrated how a school counselor made use of much of the information presented in this chapter.

CHAPTER RESOURCES

National Institute on Drug Abuse (NIDA)
www.nida.nih.gov

This website contains many great resources on drug abuse for school professionals, teachers, students, and parents.

Substance Abuse and Mental Health Services Administration (SAMHSA)
www.samhsa.gov

This website also offers lots of great resources, especially on the relation between substance abuse and mental health.

National Clearinghouse for Alcohol and Drug Information (NCADI)
ncadi.samhsa.gov

This website provides access to many resources (most of which are free) that can be ordered, including national study results, pamphlets, videos, posters, curricula, and many others.

National Institute on Alcohol Abuse and Alcoholism (NIAAA)
www.niaaa.nih.gov

This website contains information specifically related to alcohol use and abuse.

National Institute of Mental Health (NIMH)
www.nimh.nih.gov

This website provides lots of good information covering the full spectrum of mental health disorders.

Monitoring the Future (MTF)
www.nida.nih.gov

This website gives specific information on the national prevalence of substance use among students in grades 8, 10, and 12. (*Note*: Links to MTF are available on the NIDA website, as NIDA funds this ongoing research.)

National Survey on Drug Use and Health (NSDUH)
oas.samhsa.gov/nhsda.htm

This site provides national data on substance abuse and mental health issues for adolescents (ages 12–17) and adults.

42 CFR
www.lac.org/pubs/gratis.html

You can find the complete text of the regulations at this site.

FERPA
www.ed.gov/policy/gen/reg/ferpa/index.html

You can find the complete text of the regulations, and other related information, at this site.

2

Development and Maintenance of Substance Abuse

One of the questions we are frequently asked by school personnel is "Why do some students use and abuse substances, while others do not?" We wish there was a straightforward, simple answer to this question; however, the development of substance abuse depends on a variety of factors. In this chapter, we provide information on the most relevant theories of substance abuse related to student populations. Specifically, we cover the following three perspectives: biological, social learning, and risk–protective factors. We provide the most coverage of risk and protective factors in this chapter, because the theory involving these factors is the basis for many school-based substance abuse prevention and intervention programs. Thus we feel that spending more time on this particular theory will provide a greater understanding of the substance abuse prevention and intervention programs school mental health professionals are likely to encounter.

WHY DO SOME STUDENTS ABUSE SUBSTANCES?

In Chapter 1, we have indicated that many students experiment with substances without actually developing a substance abuse problem. Therefore, what makes some students more susceptible than others to abusing substances? Do some students have a biological predisposition toward substance abuse? Do some students come from environments in which they have learned that using substances is a coping mechanism? Should school mental health professionals be aware of important factors that place students at greater risk for substance abuse, or other factors that protect students from it? These represent some of the questions we are most frequently asked by school mental health professionals about student substance abuse; however, no easy answers to them exist. In order to begin trying to answer these types of questions, let us examine how the major theories attempt to explain why certain individuals are more likely to abuse substances.

BIOLOGICALLY BASED THEORIES OF SUBSTANCE ABUSE

One of the things commonly said about substance abuse is "It runs in families." For example, many people believe that a child who has an alcoholic parent is at higher risk for also acquiring an alcohol problem than a child from a family in which neither parent drinks. In fact, many of us have observed this phenomenon within families in our communities, or possibly even within our own families. These types of observations lead people to believe that substance abuse is due to some biological predisposition, inherent disorder, or disease. In order to determine the validity of such ideas, we need to examine how biological theories explain why individuals abuse substances. Generally speaking, biologically based theories of substance abuse are concerned with examining the interaction of the brain and drugs, as well as with understanding how genetics influence substance use behavior among family members. First, however, we describe a model that serves as the foundation for most of these theories.

The Disease Model

One of the most popular and long-standing theories of substance abuse is the *disease model*. This model is based on the premise that individuals abuse substances because they have an underlying disease—that is, the disease of addiction. This model gained much popularity from the work of E. M. Jellinek (1952, 1960), who proposed that alcoholism is a disease within the person. His progressive disease model of alcoholism described the stages an alcoholic person goes through, beginning with the initial drinking stage and ending with the person's experiencing a loss of control over alcohol. In fact, this loss of control is a defining feature of alcoholism, according to Jellinek's model. Furthermore, he argued that if alcoholism is a disease, then it should be treated as such; in fact, it should be regarded as a chronic and incurable condition, similar to diabetes. Therefore, the treatment of alcoholism must include strategies to manage the disease throughout a person's life.

A well-known organization that uses the disease model to help people with alcohol problems is Alcoholics Anonymous (AA). The goal of AA is for its members to maintain abstinence from alcohol, with the understanding that they will always be in the process of recovering from the addiction (AA, 2006). If you have known people in AA, you have probably heard them say such things as "I'm a recovering alcoholic" and "I'm taking things one day at a time." Statements such as these carry the underlying message that the persons view their alcoholism as a chronic problem in their lives. In fact, you have probably never heard an AA member talk about being "cured" of the disease of alcoholism. From the AA/disease model perspective, alcoholism is not a curable disease, and AA teaches its members that they will need to manage this disease on a daily basis for the rest of their lives.

The disease model is not limited to alcohol; it has also been applied to other drugs of abuse, such as cocaine and heroin (O'Brian et al., 2005). This model has also been influential in promoting biologically based research on substance abuse. For example, the disease model serves as the basis for theories about the relationships between the brain and drugs, as well as about the genetic links of substance abuse. We now examine these biologically based theories in more detail.

Brain Chemistry

It has been well established that individuals who abuse a substance actually alter their brain chemistry, and that this alteration produces experiences of euphoria and subsequent craving for the drug. Researchers who study this aspect of substance abuse examine the changes that take place within the brain after the use of particular substances. The brain is composed of billions of neurons that are used to communicate between its many parts. These neurons are very close together but do not touch; instead, they use chemical messengers called *neurotransmitters* to communicate with each other. There are many different types of neurotransmitters, which are related to the various functions regulated by the brain (e.g., experiencing pleasure, detecting pain, sleeping, eating).

One neurotransmitter that has been studied extensively in relation to substance abuse is *dopamine*. Dopamine is found in the central nervous system (CNS; i.e., the brain and spinal cord) and has been linked to such things as mood regulation, experiences of pleasure and reward, and motivation (Abadinsky, 2004). In general, drugs of abuse affect the CNS by increasing the levels of dopamine in specific brain regions, such as the *medial forebrain bundle* (Abadinsky, 2004; O'Brian et al., 2005). This brain region contains what are commonly known as the *reward pathways*. The stimulation of reward pathways produces pleasurable sensations for individuals, such as the feeling of satisfaction after eating a good meal. However, drugs of abuse also stimulate the reward pathways that produce these pleasurable sensations by increasing the levels of dopamine in this brain region (O'Brian et al., 2005). Thus behavior that results in rewards (e.g., eating, taking substances) is typically remembered and subsequently repeated because of the pleasure that it produces.

Researchers generally believe that the powerful effects of increased dopamine levels in the brain's reward pathways play a major role in the experience of dependence that individuals develop when they abuse substances over long periods of time (O'Brian et al., 2005). After the repeated use of a substance, individuals generally experience symptoms of withdrawal (e.g., negative mood, anxiety, body aches) during periods of no use. However, an individual quickly learns that taking the drug again can replace the unpleasant withdrawal symptoms with euphoria. Thus the process of experiencing euphoria and then withdrawal involves an interaction between neurotransmitters and substances of abuse (O'Brian et al., 2005). The research on brain chemistry helps us to understand this interaction; however, we still have not addressed such questions as "Are some people more susceptible to substance abuse than others?" and "Is there a genetic connection between parental substance abuse and children's use of substances?" These are important questions, and in order to address them, we now examine some of the major genetic factors related to substance abuse.

Genetic Factors

Genetically based theories of substance abuse typically revolve around the idea that the genes a child inherits from the parents contain information that can influence later substance use behavior. Genetic theories answer such questions as "Does alcoholism run in families?", "Is a child more susceptible to abusing a drug if his or her parents also abuse the drug?", or "How much can substance abuse be explained by genetics versus the environment?" In general, children of parents who abuse alcohol or other drugs are more likely to use or abuse substances than children from families in which neither parent abuses substances (Dowieko, 2002; Merikangas, Dierker, & Szatmari, 1998). Researchers have estimated that children who have alcoholic parents are three to nine times more likely to experience problems with alcohol than are children of nonalcoholic parents (Sher, 1991; Windle, 1999). In particular, sons of alcoholic fathers have been found to be four to nine times more likely to experience alcohol problems than sons of nonalcoholic fathers (Cloninger, Bohman, & Sigvardsson, 1981). After comparing a number of studies, Pollock, Schneider, Gabrielli, and Goodwin (1987) found that both males and females with alcoholism were more likely to have fathers than mothers who also had alcoholism. They also found that females with alcoholism were more likely than males to have alcoholic mothers. Studying a large sample of adopted individuals, Cloninger and colleagues (1981) found that children whose biological parents had alcoholism were more likely to develop alcoholism than were children with nonalcoholic parents. Interestingly, the children of alcoholic parents had a higher likelihood of alcoholism than the children with nonalcoholic parents, even when they were raised in families without an alcoholic adoptive parent. Taken together, the results from the studies described above suggest that children who have at least one biological parent with a substance abuse problem are at greater risk for developing substance problems of their own.

We next examine the extent to which substance abuse can be explained by genetics versus the environment. Researchers have approached this question largely by studying twins. Monozygotic or identical twins share 100% of their genes, whereas dizygotic or fraternal twins share 50% of their genes (Kendler, 2001). It is expected, then, that if a disease has a genetic component, it will occur more frequently in identical than in fraternal twins. The results of twin studies suggest that genetic factors explain 30–70% of alcohol abuse (Kendler, 2001; van den Bree, Johnson, Neale, & Pickens, 1998). Heath and Martin (1988) found in a study of young adult twins that the extent to which alcohol use could be explained by genetics differed by gender. Specifically, they found that genetics explained 47% of male alcohol use but only 35% of female alcohol use. Similarly, the influence of genetics has been used to explain the use and abuse of tobacco and illicit drugs (Sullivan & Kendler, 1999; Tsuang, Bar, Harley, & Lyons, 2001). Overall, genetic factors are thought to explain approximately 50% of the reasons why individuals use or abuse substances (O'Brian et al., 2005). What about the other 50%? To answer this question, we now turn to the environmental factors that influence the use and abuse of substances.

SOCIAL LEARNING THEORY OF SUBSTANCE ABUSE

Social Learning, Behavioral, and Cognitive-Behavioral Theories

Social learning theory is based on the premise that individuals learn things within the context of their environments through observing others (Bandura, 1977b). Specifically, this learning is believed to occur by such means as watching others model particular behaviors, seeing another person being reinforced for these behaviors, and having particular thoughts/beliefs about the behaviors being modeled (Rotgers, 2003). Social learning theory has its origins in two other psychosocial theories of substance abuse, *behavioral* and *cognitive-behavioral*. These theories are based on the premises that behavior is learned, and that a person continues or does not continue to engage in a behavior as a result of experiencing either reward or punishment for the behavior (Rotgers, 2003). Social learning theory can be considered an extension of behavioral and cognitive-behavioral theories, in that it also includes such things as observational modeling and people's thoughts/beliefs about engaging in behaviors. For the sake of simplicity, we confine the present discussion to social learning theory; however, it is important to understand that social learning theory also incorporates concepts from behavioral and cognitive-behavioral theories.

According to social learning theory, individuals can learn a range of different behaviors within the context of their environments. More specifically, individuals can learn ways to cope with challenging situations from the models (e.g., parents) in their environments. For example, most people can display a range of coping behaviors when faced with stressful situations in their environment. Many of these coping behaviors lead to positive outcomes, such as solving the problem at hand; however, individuals also learn coping behaviors that lead to negative outcomes, such as using substances to escape a stressful situation temporarily.

Substance Use as a Coping Skill

To make social learning theory and its relation to substance abuse clearer, let's consider some examples. As human beings, we are all faced with unpleasant or stressful situations as part of our daily lives. For example, sometimes we argue with family members, have a bad day at work, or get a traffic ticket (not very often, let's hope!). In order to deal with these situations, most of us have a range of *coping skills* at our disposal that we have learned. Let's think for a moment about which coping skills we use on a regular basis and how we learned them. Such coping skills can include things like telling ourselves, "Tomorrow will be a better day at work," or engaging in exercise to relieve the stresses of the day. Adolescents, however, are more likely than adults to have a limited set of coping skills, because they are in an earlier stage of development. The good news is that most adolescents respond to stressful situations in their lives by using coping skills that lead to positive outcomes. However, some adolescents rely on inferior coping skills that lead to negative outcomes, such as using substances.

Now let's imagine that a 16-year-old adolescent male named Alex has just had an argument with his parents (not a difficult situation to imagine for anyone who works with or has adolescents!). After the argument, Alex feels angry, is upset, and does not want to be around his parents, so he retreats to his room. From past experiences, Alex has learned that when he feels angry, he is able to feel better by smoking marijuana. He subsequently smokes a joint of marijuana in his room, with his window open and a blanket at the bottom of his door to ensure that his parents will not smell it. After smoking the marijuana, Alex does in fact feel better. His anger has dissipated; in fact, he cannot even remember why he was arguing with his parents. For adolescents who use substances as a coping behavior, this type of scenario is not uncommon. One of us (Burrow-Sanchez) has worked with adolescents in substance abuse treatment who have described similar ways of dealing with arguments with their parents. From this example, it is not difficult to see how an adolescent can quickly develop a substance problem by learning that after every argument with a parent (i.e., stressful situation), he or she feels better after smoking marijuana (i.e., coping skill).

Modeling

One researcher who has had a significant influence on the development of social learning theory is Albert Bandura. In particular, his work on *modeling* has taught us many things about the ways in which individuals learn from each other. As mentioned above, children, adolescents, and adults can learn behaviors (both good and bad) from observing models in their environments (Bandura, 1977b). In addition, a person is more likely to imitate a model if the model is similar to him or her (e.g., a same-sex parent or peer). Thus it is not difficult to imagine how children learn behaviors from their parents; examples might include a little girl imitating her mother while she is putting on makeup before work, or a little boy with a toy lawn mower imitating his father mowing the yard. Some children and adolescents learn behaviors through the process of modeling that leads to negative outcomes. Let's return to the case of Alex. Alex has often observed his father come home after a day of work at a demanding and stressful job, and drink a few cocktails before and during dinner to "relieve stress," as his father puts it. Alex's father is thus modeling the use of a substance (i.e., alcohol) as an appropriate way to deal with stress. Clearly, this situation is very similar to Alex's use of marijuana to deal with his anger after having an argument with his parents. Of course, the process of modeling is not restricted to the family environment, and we could have also described an example involving one of Alex's peers instead of his father.

Self-Efficacy Expectations

There is an additional component of social learning theory that we want to address briefly. Bandura (1977a, 1994) has also taught us that individuals have beliefs about their ability to perform behaviors, which he terms *self-efficacy expectations*. What this means is that we are more likely to try behaviors that we think we can do and will lead to successful outcomes (i.e., behaviors for which we have high self-efficacy), in contrast to behaviors that we think we may not be able to do and may produce negative outcomes (i.e., behaviors for which we have low self-efficacy). For example, when an individual learns a behavior from a model, it does not guarantee that the individual will attempt the behavior. Thus the individual also needs to believe that he or she can carry out a similar behavior and that it will lead to positive outcomes. Related to this, self-efficacy for behavior can also be learned through the individual's direct experiences while engaging in the behavior.

To make this clearer, let's again return to the example of Alex. Now imagine that Alex previously attempted to use a better coping skill (e.g., negotiation) during arguments with his parents. That is, he tried negotiating with his parents during two prior arguments, but quickly learned that he still did not get what he wanted and continued to feel angry afterward. Based on his past experiences, Alex has come to believe that negotiating with his parents during an argument is not a very useful strategy. In contrast, Alex has learned that smoking marijuana after arguments with his parents makes him feel much better about the situation; consequently, smoking marijuana has become a preferred coping skill for Alex. The point we want to highlight here is that although adolescents can learn positive coping skills for managing stressful situations (e.g., negotiation), such coping skills are not likely to be used if the adolescents believe that the skills will not be effective in dealing with a situation (i.e., low self-efficacy), and thus they are more likely to use coping skills that they see as producing more positive outcomes (i.e., high self-efficacy).

We have now described from a social learning theory perspective how adolescents can learn particular behaviors within their environments. However, such questions as "Why do some adolescents use and abuse substances, while others do not?" and "How do the environments of adolescents who abuse substances differ from those of adolescents who do not?" have still not been fully addressed. We take up these questions in the next section. As noted at the beginning of the chapter, our discussion of risk and protective factors is more detailed than our earlier discussions, as this area is likely to serve as the basis for many school-based prevention and intervention programs.

RISK AND PROTECTIVE FACTORS
FOR STUDENT SUBSTANCE ABUSE

Ecology of Risk and Protective Factors

Prior to providing a description of specific risk and protective factors, we want to establish an environmental context for this information. More specifically, Bronfenbrenner (1979) suggested that human development should be conceptualized within the context of the environments that influence it. According to Bronfenbrenner, humans develop within an ecology composed of many different domains or environments that operate at many different levels throughout the life span. For example, a child is born with individual characteristics (e.g., temperament), which develop in relation to the influences from his or her proximal environment (e.g., family) or more distal environment (e.g., state laws). To make this clearer, Figure 2.1 presents an ecological model of how a child's development is influenced by the many domains operating at different levels. The

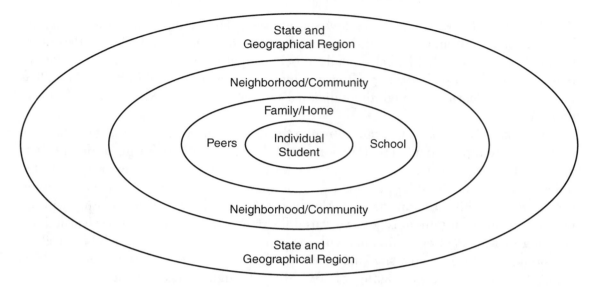

FIGURE 2.1. Ecological model of development.

domains closer to the individual student (i.e., family, school, peers) have more direct influence, whereas the more distal domains (e.g., state and geographical region) exert influence in less direct ways (e.g., state laws). As you read the following discussion of specific risk and protective factors, consider which domain(s) these factors fit into, as well as how they can influence the student at multiple levels.

Defining Risk and Protective Factors

Regardless of the specific theory of substance abuse they endorse, most researchers agree on the influence of risk and protective factors on the development of substance abuse in children and adolescents (Benman, 1995; Clayton, 1992; Hawkins, Catalano, & Miller, 1992; Weinburg, 2001). A *risk factor* is typically defined as anything that increases the probability of a person using drugs, whereas a *protective factor* is anything that decreases this probability (Clayton, 1992). For example, a risk factor for substance abuse is having a parent with a drug abuse problem, and a protective factor is high academic achievement in school. Risk and protective factors are found in all domains of an adolescent's life (e.g., school, family, peers) and are influenced by variables such as age, gender, and ethnicity (Hawkins et al., 1992; Moon, Hecht, Jackson, & Spellers, 1999; Vega & Gil, 1998). In general, the higher the number of risk factors for a given adolescent, the greater his or her risk will be for developing substance abuse problems. In contrast, protective factors act to increase an adolescent's ability to resist pressures to use or abuse substances. Although no single protective factor has been shown to prevent drug use, the higher the quantity and quality of protective factors present, the stronger the effect they will have on limiting an adolescent's drug use (Newcomb, 1995).

Major Categories of Risk and Protective Factors

Hawkins and his colleagues (1992) initially described many risk and protective factors for adolescent substance abuse, and their description has been expanded on upon in recent years. These factors can be categorized into five major domains of an adolescent's life: individual, peer, family, school, and community. We present a comprehensive list of risk and protective factors in Table 2.1 for each domain and we now discuss these factors by domain in greater detail.

Individual Factors

Individual factors are intrapersonal characteristics of the adolescent (which are either learned or inherited). One individual risk factor for substance abuse is exhibiting problem behaviors from an early age, such as previous drug use, aggressiveness toward others, negative moods, withdrawal, and/or impulsivity. Another is having a coexisting mental health diagnosis, such as conduct disorder, attention-deficit/hyperactivity disorder (ADHD), depression, or a learning disorder. Certain individual risk factors can be the targets of intervention (e.g., poor social skills), whereas others cannot be (e.g., an adolescent's genetic predisposition). It is also worthy to note that many of these factors not only place a student at higher risk for substance abuse, but are also risk factors for other problems, such as disruptive behavior and delinquency. Furthermore, as noted in Chapter 1, other disorders such as depression and ADHD frequently co-occur with substance abuse (Riggs, 2003). Thus it is important to understand the time line for each disorder, as an adolescent may be using substances to "self-medicate" for the co-occurring disorder. Substance use or abuse may even be a symptom of another underlying disorder.

Researchers have also identified individual protective factors that work to buffer adolescents from developing problems with drugs. Many protective factors (but not all) are essentially the opposites of risk factors. For example, a risk factor for adolescent substance abuse is deficits in problem solving, whereas a protective factor is good problem-solving ability. That said, individual protective factors include good social and problem-solving skills, lack of mental health disorders, and positive perceptions of self-worth (i.e., high self-esteem) (Hawkins et al., 1992; Newcomb, 1995). Therefore, good mental health is a protective factor against substance abuse as well as many other problems and disorders.

Peer Factors

The second major domain of risk and protective factors for adolescent substance abuse is the peer group. The period of adolescence is a time when the influence of one's peer group becomes more pronounced; in relation to substance abuse, peer groups are particularly important. For example, adolescents who associate with drug-using peers have consistently been found to have higher levels of drug use (Barnes & Welte, 1986; Kandel & Andrews, 1987; Weber, Graham, Hansen, Flay, & Johnston, 1989). In fact, our typical

TABLE 2.1. Risk and Protective Factors for Adolescent Substance Use and Abuse

Domain	Risk factors	Protective factors
Individual	• Early age at first use • Deficits in social skills and problem solving • Early and persistent behavioral acting out • Hostility and aggression • Impulsivity • Learning disabilities • Alienation • Rebelliousness • Physical trauma • Favorable attitudes toward use • Genetic predisposition for drug use • Mental health disorders (e.g., depression)	• Good social skills and problem solving • Good mental health • Emotional stability • Positive sense of self (e.g., self-esteem, self-worth) • Flexibility • Resiliency
Peers	• Peers who use or abuse drugs • Peers with favorable attitudes toward drug use • Peers who engage in delinquent behavior • Peer rejection • Peers with deficits in social skills and problem solving	• Peers who engage in prosocial activities (e.g., academics, sports) • Peers with negative attitudes toward drug use • Peers with social competency: —Social skills —Problem solving —Assertiveness • Peers with good communication skills
Family	• Parent(s) or older sibling(s) who use/abuse drugs • Family member(s) with favorable attitudes toward drug use • High conflict or stress in family • Low bonding to parents and/or family • Poor parenting practices: —Low monitoring —Inconsistent and harsh discipline —Poor problem solving —Low levels of parental support • Parent(s) with mental health problems (e.g., depression)	• Effective parenting practices: —Appropriate monitoring —High expectations —Clear rules and expectations —Appropriate levels of support (e.g., emotional) • Positive bonding to family • Sense of trust within family
School	• Academic failure • Low commitment or bonding to school • Inappropriate classroom behavior (e.g., withdrawn, overly aggressive) • Low teacher expectations • School disorganization • Unsafe school climate • Unclear school policies on drug use	• Participation, involvement, and responsibility in: —School tasks —School decisions • Safe and supportive school climate • High expectations by school personnel • School with clear standards and rules for appropriate behavior
Community	• Norms favoring substance use • Disorganized and unsafe neighborhoods: —High crime —High poverty —Lack of community resources —Lack of physical maintenance (e.g., run-down buildings, streets, and homes) • High levels of family transition and mobility • Disenfranchised cultural groups	• Safe and supportive community • High standards and expectations for youth • Positive community-based activities readily available (e.g., at churches, youth centers) • Positive community-sponsored activities available (e.g., celebrations, festivals) • Education about positive and negative media influences

Note. This table is based on the following sources: Alberta Alcohol and Drug Abuse Commission (2003); Hawkins, Catalano, and Miller (1992); Newcomb (1995); Robertson, David, and Rao (2003).

response to the common question "How do you know if a student is using substances?" is "Does he or she spend time with friends who use drugs?" If the answer is yes, then there is a high likelihood that the student is also using or has at least tried drugs. One of us (Burrow-Sanchez) has had many discussions with adolescent clients in substance abuse treatment about the influence of their peers, and many of these adolescents have stated frankly that their level of drug use would probably be less if they did not have friends who also used. At this point, it may seem that a simple solution is just to ask such students to associate with peers who do not use substances. In practice, this is much easier said than done, and many adolescent clients have balked at the idea. Changing one's peer group is a difficult task for anyone; for example, think about how hard it would be for you to stop interacting with all of your close friends. From clinical experience, Burrow-Sanchez has found that it is generally more productive when working with adolescents to discuss the influence of their peer group and then brainstorm ways to lessen negative peer influences, such as spending less time with drug-using peers or avoiding locations where peers use drugs. More specific strategies for one-to-one work with students are presented in Chapter 5.

Peers also influence adolescent behavior and attitudes in many positive ways. Peers who do not use drugs and have negative attitudes toward the use of substances are likely to influence similar behavior and attitudes in an adolescent (Hawkins et al., 1992). In addition, an adolescent whose peer group engages in prosocial activities (e.g., sports or school government) is also more likely to engage in socially sanctioned activities. This does not mean that students whose peers have negative attitudes about drug use and engage in prosocial behaviors will never try drugs. In fact, it is likely that most adolescents will try substances at some point prior to graduating from high school (see Chapter 1 for adolescent use statistics). One study even found that adolescents who experimented with substances were more psychologically healthy than adolescents who never tried substances (Shelder & Block, 1990). Thus one could argue that experimentation with substances is part of typical adolescent development, as the majority of adolescents who experiment with substances will not go on to develop a substance abuse problem (Newcomb, 1995; Shelder & Block, 1990). As we have discussed, adolescence is a time when one's peer group begins to have more influence; however, the family system continues to influence the adolescent throughout his or her development. We now turn to examining specific risk and protective factors within the family domain.

Family Factors

The third major domain of risk and protective factors for adolescent substance abuse is the family. Most of us like to believe that families nurture and support their children to develop into healthy adults. In general, most families do provide a context for the healthy development of their children. Some students, however, come from families that put them at risk for the use and abuse of substances. Our example above involving Alex can help us illustrate one of the family-based risk factors. More specifically, the research evidence indicates that the risk of using drugs increases when an adolescent has a parent or older sibling who uses drugs (Brook, Whiteman, Gordon, & Brook, 1990; Johnson, Schoutz, & Locke, 1984), and this has been shown in the case of Alex.

Several identifiable poor parenting practices have also been consistently linked to many negative outcomes for children, including substance abuse and delinquent behavior (Hawkins et al., 1992). More specifically, parenting practices such as low levels of parental supervision for children, use of inconsistent and harsh discipline tactics, poor display of problem-solving skills, and low levels of emotional support provided to children are linked to negative psychological and behavior outcomes for children. High levels of marital conflict or family stress also place children at risk for negative outcomes such as substance abuse (Hawkins et al., 1992). It is not difficult to imagine that a child who comes from a family in which poor parenting practices are combined with high levels of marital distress will have a low level of bonding to his or her family. In fact, low levels of bonding to the family unit is itself another risk factor for adolescent substance abuse. In addition, the children of parents who experience mental health problems, such as depression, are at higher risk for mental health problems than are children with mentally healthy parents (Cummings & Davies, 1999). Poor parental mental health is a particularly strong risk factor for many negative outcomes for children, especially when the parents do not obtain appropriate treatment for their disorders. As suggested above, the transference of mental health problems from parents to children is a process that has both genetic and environmental components.

In contrast to the poor parenting practices described above, positive parenting practices promote good outcomes for children and adolescents. These practices include such things as appropriate levels of child monitoring, setting clear rules and expectations for children, and expressing high levels of emotional support to children. The use of positive parenting practices can lead to the development of strong bonds and trust between an adolescent and his or her family, which is another protective factor against substance abuse. It probably goes without saying that parents' lack of substance use is a protective factor against adolescent substance use or abuse, as are negative parental attitudes toward the use of substances.

Even though peer groups become more important during the period of adolescence, parents still have much influence on their adolescents' behavior. For example, unfavorable parental attitudes toward the use of drugs are related to unfavorable adolescent attitudes toward drug use and lower levels of actual drug use (Hawkins et al., 1992). Recent data from the National Study on Drug Use and Health (NSDUH) indicated that adolescents ages 12–17 who were less likely to use drugs also perceived that their parents would strongly disapprove of drug use (SAMHSA, 2003). More specifically, of the 89.1% of adolescents who perceived that their parents would strongly disapprove of using marijuana, only 5.5% had used it in the past month (SAMHSA, 2003). Therefore, these data suggest that parental views of drug use influence their children's drug use attitudes and actual drug use behavior. Outside of the family, the largest socializing agent for children and adolescents is the school environment. We now turn to a discussion of school-based risk and protective factors.

School Factors

One consistent finding is that students who abuse substances also generally experience academic and behavioral failure at school (Hawkins et al., 1992). Such students also have low commitments to school and view it as a negative place because they experience unpleasant consequences such as detention or suspension. It is important to note that these students are also at risk for dropping out of school (Clayton, 1992). In fact, as noted in Chapter 1, students who drop out of school are more likely than those who stay in school to use substances (Mensch & Kandel, 1988). Another risk factor that teachers frequently observe is inappropriate classroom behavior, such as either excessive aggression toward others or excessive withdrawal. In general, the younger the age at which a student displays such disruptive or withdrawn behaviors, the more negative the later substance-abuse-related outcomes are (Hawkins et al., 1992).

In addition to observable behaviors in students, certain school characteristics are risk factors in themselves. For example, schools that have low expectations for students, are disorganized and unsafe, or do not have clear expectations regarding appropriate student behavior place students at higher risk for substance abuse and other problem behaviors (Mayer, 1995; Skiba & Peterson, 1999; Sugai, Horner, & Gresham, 2002). It is not difficult to see that school-related risk factors occur on multiple levels, which include the individual student, school personnel, and schoolwide characteristics.

As most of our readers already know, schools can also be a great source of protective factors for students. Even when a student comes from a difficult home environment, the school setting can provide protective factors that greatly reduce the risk for many problem behaviors. In order for the school to be a protective factor, the student needs to have a strong bond or connection to it. In part, positive connections are built when students become involved in school activities that lead to positive outcomes, such as participating in sports, clubs, or committees. In addition, students who have good academic achievement generally have much more positive attitudes and bonds to school than students who are at risk for academic failure (Clayton, 1992).

Characteristics of the schoolwide environment can also serve as protective factors against student substance abuse. These include clear standards for appropriate student behavior that are known to all school personnel and students. For example, many schools across the nation have adopted a schoolwide positive behavior support plan, which includes setting up common expectations or "rules" for appropriate student behavior (Colvin, Kame'enui, & Sugai, 1993; Walker et al., 1996). Schools decide on three to five positively stated expectations, such as "Be Responsible," "Be Respectful," and "Hands and Feet to Self," and teach students what these expectations should look like in specific settings around the school. For example, to "Be Respectful" in a middle school cafeteria involves students' waiting their turn in line for lunch, asking politely for the food choices they desire, and following the directions of the adults who are supervising the cafeteria. Examples of *not* being respectful in this situation are given as well. Schools actively teach these expectations during the first week of school and provide boosters and reminders throughout the year. Schools also develop a schoolwide reinforcement plan to acknowledge students who are following the expectations. For more information on how to implement a schoolwide behavior support plan, see Taylor-Greene and colleagues (1997) or the website of the National Technical Assistance Center on Positive Behavioral Interventions and Supports (*www.pbis.org*).

Finally, schools can provide safe physical environments and supportive climates, which serve as protective factors for all students. Examples include regularly maintaining buildings on campus, students feeling safe at school, and school personnel fostering a climate of support for student achievement.

Community Factors

The last major domain consists of risk and protective factors in the community and neighborhood. We define *communities* as large social environments such as cities or towns, which are composed of many smaller social environments called *neighborhoods*. However, for the sake of simplicity, we discuss both community and neighborhood factors here as "community." We also include some factors in this discussion that, strictly speaking, would fall into the "State and Georgraphical Region" area of Figure 2.1. Community factors in this broader sense include such things as geographical characteristics, local and state laws, socioeconomic status (SES), population density, crime rates, and attitudes toward substance use.

Community risk factors for adolescent substance abuse include adult and community norms that favor drug use, lax drug laws, and high availability of drugs. For example, lower legal drinking ages and lower taxation of alcohol are risk factors for use and abuse of alcohol in a given geographical region. When the legal age of drinking is increased, fewer alcohol-related traffic incidents are reported (Saffer & Grossman, 1987). Similarly, higher taxation of alcohol in a geographical area is related to overall decreases in consumption (Levy & Sheflin, 1985; Saffer & Grossman, 1987). Another influential community risk factor is the availability of drugs, which tends to vary across communities, depending on the laws of the city or state and the local norms regarding drug use. In general, the more available drugs are in a given community, the more likely it is that adolescents will report using them (Gorsuch & Butler, 1976; Maddahian, Newcomb, & Bentler, 1988). In fact, data from the NSDUH indicate that more than 50% of adolescents ages 12–17 consider marijuana "fairly" or "very" easy to acquire in their communities (SAMHSA, 2003).

Additional community factors that create risk for adolescent substance abuse are disorganized and unsafe neighborhoods (Hawkins et al., 1992; Newcomb, 1995). In such neighborhoods, residents do not feel as if they have a sense of "community." Factors that contribute to disorganization and lack of safety include high crime, poverty, and a general failure to maintain commercial buildings and homes. In addition, families in some of the poorest communities in our nation have a high level of mobility, which leads to an unstable community environment. For instance, members of immigrant families may move frequently, depending on the availability of work in a geographical region.

Individuals from racial and ethnic minority groups (e.g., Mexican American, African American) in our nation generally experience higher rates of poverty than individuals from the European American population, as indicated by U.S. Bureau of the Census (2004) data. In part, the poverty experienced by individuals from racial and ethnic minority groups serves to segregate communities in most large cities based on socioeconomic status. For example, the city in which we authors live is socioeconomically divided into the "West" and "East" sides. Many people with lower SES live on the "West" side of the city, whereas individuals living on the "East" side are of relatively higher SES. Furthermore, larger numbers of individuals from racial and ethnic minority groups (largely Hispanic) live on the "West" side, whereas the "East" side is mostly inhabited by European Americans. The point we are making is that racial and ethnic minority groups can easily feel disenfranchised from the larger community in which they live, due to both geographical and socioeconomic segregation. In addition, the attitudes, feelings, and behaviors associated with this disenfranchisement can serve as a risk factor for adolescent substance abuse.

In contrast to the community risk factors we have just described above, many protective factors can be provided by communities. These protective factors can include safe environments for residents, high standards for young people, and a range of positive community activities for residents (Hawkins et al., 1992; Newcomb, 1995). In particular, strong and positive bonds to the community serve as a protective factor against drug abuse and other problem behaviors for adolescents. Adolescents can build strong bonds to their communities by participating in prosocial community-based activities at such venues as youth centers (e.g., Boys and Girls Clubs), churches, and other positive socializing agents. In general, adolescents who feel positive connections to their communities are less at risk for substance abuse than adolescents who do not.

CASE EXAMPLE

Amy, a school psychologist at Hill Valley Middle School for 5 years, was quite adept at assessing students for intellectual functioning and learning disabilities. Because of her expertise, she was frequently contacted by other school personnel (e.g., teachers, counselors) for consultation on students. Recently she was contacted by a teacher in her school, who indicated that a new student named Ray had recently transferred from another school into her classroom. The teacher was concerned because Ray seemed to be withdrawn and reserved during class; for example, he rarely participated in class discussions and had minimal interactions with other students outside of class. The teacher reported that his past school record indicated mediocre grades and no evidence of any learning problems. However, the teacher reported that Ray did not seem to be "getting" the material in her class, and that he was not working at grade level. At first the teacher thought that Ray's behavior was due to his being a new transfer student, and she assumed that he would adjust to his new school within a few weeks. After 2 months, however, Ray's behavior had not improved; in fact, he seemed even more withdrawn. When the teacher spoke with Ray about his class performance, she stated that he appeared a bit "out of it" and "spaced out." She also reported that his demeanor seemed overly calm and that he appeared not to take anything too seriously. The teacher feared that if Ray's performance did not improve, he would fail her class. The teacher also wondered whether Ray might have a learning disorder that had been overlooked by his previous school. Thus the teacher referred Ray to Amy to rule out the presence of any learning disorders.

Amy set up a meeting with Ray to assess this possibility. At the start of this meeting, Amy learned that he had recently transferred to the school because of his parents' divorce a few months earlier. Ray's mother had full custody of him and his 16-year old brother; their father visited the two of them every other weekend. Furthermore, Ray's mom had moved him and his brother to Hill Valley (which was 60 miles away from his previous school) in order to make a "fresh start." Ray stated that the move had been "okay" except for his having to change schools and leave his old friends behind. He reported that his parents "always fought," so he could understand why they got divorced and why they still did not get along. Ray described his father as "always drinking," and he noted that this was the cause of a lot of his parents' arguments. Ray also stated that his older brother was in high school and frequently "smoked pot." Ray said that his brother hid his pot smoking from their mother; however, Ray thought that his mother knew about it but just did not say anything. He said that his mother probably would not care about his older brother's pot use as long as he stayed in school and out of trouble.

Ray said that before the divorce he had worried a lot about how things would turn out for his family. He admitted that he really had not wanted his parents to split up, even though they argued frequently. He said the divorce and subsequent move to a new town and school had been difficult for him and was "a lot to deal with." Amy asked Ray what things he had been doing to deal with the situation, and he responded, "I've found some things to help me deal with it." Ray was hesitant to explain further about his ways of "dealing with it," and Amy did not push him. The remainder of this initial meeting consisted of Amy's administering tests to assess Ray for a learning disorder. The initial meeting was not long enough to complete the testing, so a second meeting was scheduled.

A week later, Amy met with Ray to finish the testing. Still curious, Amy asked Ray how he had been "dealing with things" since the last time they saw each other. Ray stated that he had been "dealing with things okay," but that his mom had been "on my case" because she found out that he was smoking marijuana. Ray was surprisingly open about his marijuana use and said that he began using it shortly after moving from his old town, because he felt "bad" because of the divorce and loss of contact with his prior friends. In fact, he stated that he frequently came to school "high," as he would smoke marijuana in the mornings before school. He said that smoking marijuana made him feel better about the situation with his parents and his "new life" in Hill Valley. Amy then completed the testing with Ray, but (as she suspected) the results did not indicate a learning disorder.

Amy believed that the behavior observed by Ray's teacher could be explained by his marijuana use. For example, Ray had admitted that he often came to school "high," and it was his first-period teacher who had made the referral. Ray was likely to be most intoxicated during first period, before the drug had time to wear off during the day. Amy felt that Ray needed help in dealing with the divorce of his parents and his marijuana use before he could perform better in school. Hill Valley Middle School had a zero tolerance policy in effect regarding student drug use; however, Amy also knew that the administration had discretion in terms of consequences for drug use. Following the school's policies,

Amy told Ray that she had a duty to inform the administration and his mother about his drug use. She also thanked him for telling her, and she promised that she would assist him in getting the necessary help in order to deal with the divorce of his parents more effectively than by using marijuana. At first Ray was upset about Amy's having to tell anyone about his drug use, but after discussing it for a while and understanding her genuine wish to help him, he soon became more agreeable to the idea.

Although Amy was not an expert in adolescent substance use, she made a quick assessment of Ray's risk and protective factors across five domains (see Table 2.2). She quickly determined that certain risk factors were present for Ray; however, there were many protective factors present as well. In fact, Amy was hopeful that she had caught Ray's substance use in its early stages and could prevent it from becoming a more serious substance problem if he could get proper help in dealing with the divorce of his parents. Amy also knew that she could use her knowledge of risk and protective factors to advocate for Ray when she approached her school's administrators.

TABLE 2.2. Ray's Risk and Protective Factors for Substance Abuse

Domain	Risk factors	Protective factors
Individual	• Possible genetic predisposition (father's use of alcohol) • Possible depression (due to parents' recent divorce) • Withdrawal in class	• Brief history of marijuana use • No prior history of mental health disorders • No prior history of problems at school
Peers	• No peer group at new school; may gravitate toward peers who use drugs if not addressed	• Peers at old school who did not use • Not yet established with peer group at new school (important to gravitate toward positive peer group) • No apparent problems joining with a peer group at old school
Family	• Father's and older sibling's use of substances. • Recent divorce of parents; marital discord	• Parenting practices apparently sufficient (however, recently strained by divorce) • In general, good bonding with family; postdivorce situation less clear • No evidence of parental mental health disorders
School	• Recent drop in grades • Recent drop in commitment to school	• Past grades average • Past commitment to school • Present school personnel concerned about student's welfare • Present school environment with clear expectations and rules regarding student drug use
Community	• Drugs available in community (however, not more so than in average community)	• Middle-SES community • Safe and supportive community • Community with generally negative views of drug use • Many community-based activities and services available to youth • Many educational and treatment approaches available to adolescents with substance abuse problems in community

As it turned out, Ray's mother was more concerned about getting him help than about punishing him or his marijuana use. In addition, the administrators decided, in part as a result of Amy's advocacy, that Ray could benefit more from community treatment resources than from school suspension. He was subsequently referred to a psycho-educational course in the community that focused on building positive coping and problem-solving skills instead of using drugs. Amy also referred Ray to a group in the middle school, run by a school counselor, for students dealing with the divorce of their parents. Within a month or so, Ray's class performance and grades had improved, and he disclosed to Amy that he was finding more positive ways to deal with the divorce. She also noticed that his risk factors for substance abuse were less prominent than at their first meeting, and that many protective factors were being enhanced as he received the proper support in dealing with his parents' divorce.

CHAPTER SUMMARY

The reasons why adolescents use and abuse substances are varied and complex. We have discussed theories of substance abuse based on three major perspectives: biological, social learning, and risk–protective factors. Findings from studies based on biological theories such as the disease model, brain chemistry, and genetics indicate that biology plays a substantial role; for instance, approximately 50% of substance problems can be explained from a genetic perspective. The other 50% of reasons why people abuse substances are explained by environmental factors such as those proposed by social learning theory. Most relevant for school mental health professionals is the risk–protective factor theory of substance abuse. In particular, these professionals should understand which factors place students at higher or lower risk for developing substance abuse problems. Finally, a case example has illustrated how a school psychologist integrated much of the information presented in this chapter into her work with a student.

CHAPTER RESOURCES

American Council for Drug Education
www.acde.org

This website, hosted by Phoenix House, provides a lot of information and material for teens, parents, and educators on the topic of substance abuse.

National Clearinghouse for Alcohol and Drug Information (NCADI)
ncadi.samhsa.gov

This is a government-hosted website that lists thousands of resources on substance use and abuse, which can be directly ordered from the site. Most of these materials can be obtained free of charge.

National Institute on Drug Abuse (NIDA)

www.nida.nih.gov

This website has lots of great research-based information for students, parents, and school professionals regarding adolescent substance abuse. Much of this material is also available in Spanish.

NIDA for Teens

teens.drugabuse.gov/parents/index.asp

This is a website sponsored by NIDA and tailored specifically for adolescents.

Parents: The Anti-Drug

www.theantidrug.com

This website is sponsored by the National Youth Anti-Drug Media Campaign and provides information on substance abuse for parents, as well as for students and school professionals.

Social Development Research Group

depts.washington.edu/sdrg

This research group at the University of Washington has conducted much of the pioneering work on the topic of risk and protective factors for adolescent substance abuse. Browse the website to find lots of useful information.

U.S. Drug Enforcement Administration (DEA)

www.dea.gov

This site provides information on national drug control policies, as well as links to information on preventing substance abuse in youth.

3

Knowing Drugs of Abuse and Screening for a Substance Abuse Problem

In this chapter we provide information on various drugs of abuse, as well as on screening students for substance abuse problems. In our work with school mental health professionals, we are frequently asked, "How can you tell if a student is using drugs?" or "How can I tell how severe a student's drug problem really is?" We address these and similar questions throughout the course of this chapter. First, we present a description of the major drugs of abuse, because we have heard from many school mental health professionals that they want to know more about the types of drugs adolescents use. Second, we discuss the various aspects of screening for a substance abuse problem: issues of consent and confidentiality, the differences between screening and assessment, and establishing a positive working relationship with a student. Third, we provide an in-depth discussion of a four-step screening procedure that school mental health professionals can easily implement, as well as a list of available screening measures. Finally, we present a case example that illustrates the use of the material covered in this chapter. In writing this chapter, we have realized that many school mental health professionals may not feel qualified either to screen or to assess students for substance abuse. However, we also believe that many such professionals have a desire to understand at least how to screen students for substance problems. Given this, we have chosen to focus this chapter primarily on screening rather than assessment, because we want to present practices that the majority of school mental health professionals can easily implement, even if they have minimal prior training in this area.

MAJOR SUBSTANCES OF ABUSE

Drugs of abuse enter a user's body in one of the following ways: orally, via inhalation, or via injection. After entering the body, drugs are absorbed in the bloodstream and carried to the central nervous system (CNS), which is composed of the brain and spinal cord. The brain is protected by what is called the *blood–brain barrier*. This barrier protects the brain from being exposed to toxins in the bloodstream. However, drugs of abuse pass through this barrier and affect the brain by altering the balance of neurotransmitters. As noted in Chapter 2, *neurotransmitters* are chemicals that send messages between the neurons in the CNS. Not all drugs affect the CNS in the same way. For example, depressants such as alcohol slow down the CNS, whereas stimulants such as cocaine speed up the CNS. For this reason, drugs of abuse are typically categorized in terms of the effects they have on the CNS. Throughout this section of the chapter, we also use the terms *tolerance* and *withdrawal* to describe how specific drugs interact with the body. As described in greater detail in Chapter 1, *tolerance* refers to a person using more of a substance in order to obtain the same desired effect; *withdrawal* refers to a person experiencing unpleasant physical or psychological symptoms after reducing or stopping the use of a drug (American Psychiatric Association, 2000). We now describe the major categories of drugs as well as the specific substances within these categories. Table 3.1 summarizes this information.

Depressants

Depressants slow down the CNS and generally make the user feel better by lowering anxiety and reducing inhibitions. For example, people refer to alcohol as a "social lubricant" because it has these effects in situations such as social gatherings. Depressants also slow down a person's pulse, breathing, blood pressure, and other bodily functions. In fact, when depressants are taken in large amounts or mixed with one another (e.g., when alcohol and barbiturates are combined), they can shut down these functions and in extreme cases can cause death. In general, people using depressants can quickly develop tolerance to these substances. Withdrawal is also common and can be very dangerous, as it can lead to seizures and potential death; people withdrawing from depressants should be supervised by a medical professional because of the potentially lethal consequences. The category of depressants includes alcohol, barbiturates, benzodiazepines, and a few others.

Alcohol

Alcohol is the substance most commonly used by adolescents (see Chapter 1 for use statistics). This fact is not hard to believe, given that alcohol can be legally purchased by persons over 21 years of age in the United States, is readily available, and is commonly found in many adolescents' homes. The physical effects of alcohol largely depend on a

TABLE 3.1. Drugs of Abuse

Drug name	Commercial names	Common street names (slang)	Potential intoxication effects	Potential negative effects	Routes of administration
Depressants					
Alcohol (ethanol) (e.g., beer, wine, distilled liquor)	Various brand names	Various	General disinhibition, relaxation, stress reduction, euphoria; anesthesia	Depresses CNS; problems with motor activity, speech, thinking; coma or death at very high doses; adverse pregnancy outcomes (e.g., fetal alcohol syndrome)	Oral
Barbiturates	Amytal, Nembutal, Seconal, Phenobarbital	Blues, yellows, or reds; blue, yellow, or red birds; barbs; phennies	Sedation and drowsiness	Depression, unusual excitement, fever, irritability, poor judgement, slurred speech, dizziness; withdrawal can be lethal	Oral and injected
Benzodiazepines	Ativan, Halcion, Librium, Valium, Xanax	Candy, downers, sleeping pills, vals	Sedation and drowsiness	Dizziness	Oral and injected
Flunitrazepam	Rohypnol	Forget-me pill, Mexican Valium, R2, roche, roofies, roofinol, rope, rophies	Drowsiness and memory loss; can result in sexual assaults and date rape	Vision and gastrointestinal problems; urinary retention; memory loss while under the influence of the drug	Oral and snorted
Gamma-hydroxybutyrate (GHB)	N/A	G, Georgia home boy, grievous bodily harm, liquid ecstasy	Drowsiness; can result in sexual assaults and date rape	Nausea and vomiting; headache; loss of consciousness and reflexes; seizures; potential coma and death	Oral
Methaqualone	Quaalude, Sopor, Parest	Ludes, mandrex, quad, quay	Elevated sense of well-being (euphoria)	Depression, poor reflexes, slurred speech, potential coma	Oral and injected
			Common to depressants: Reduced anxiety, euphoria, disinhibition	*Common to depressants:* Decreases in pulse, breathing, and blood pressure; poor concentration; fatigue, confusion; problems with coordination, memory, and judgment; respiratory depression and arrest; overdose and withdrawal can be lethal	
Stimulants					
Amphetamines	Biphetamine, Dexedrine	Bennies, black beauties, crosses, speed, truck drivers, uppers	*Common to stimulants:* General stimulation; increased energy levels and mental alertness; feelings of exhilaration	Problems with coordination; tremor, anxiousness, nervousness, irritability, restlessness, impulsiveness, panic, paranoia; reduced appetite, weight loss; insomnia, heart failure	Oral, injected, smoked, or snorted
Methamphetamine	Desoxyn	Chalk, crank, crystal, glass, go fast, ice, meth, speed		Aggression, violence, psychotic behavior; problems with learning and memory; heart and neurological damage; reduced appetite, weight loss; insomnia, nervousness, heart failure	Oral, injected, smoked, or snorted

46

Substance	Commercial/Trade Names	Common/Street Names	Health Effects	Route of Administration
Cocaine	N/A	Blow, bump, C, candy, coke, crack, flake, nose candy, rock, snow, toot	Increased temperature; chest pain, respiratory failure, nausea, abdominal pain, strokes, seizures, headaches, malnutrition, panic attacks; reduced appetite, weight loss; insomnia, nervousness, heart failure	Snorted, smoked, or injected
Methylphenidate	Ritalin	JIF, MPH, R's, R-ball, rits, skippy, the smart drug, vitamin R	Increased heart rate, blood pressure, metabolism; reduced appetite, weight loss; insomnia, nervousness, heart failure	Oral, snorted, or injected
Nicotine (e.g., cigarettes, cigars, smokeless tobacco)	Various brand names	Cigs, cancer sticks, snuff, chew, spit	Chronic coughs and sore throats; chronic lung disease, cardiovascular disease, cancer; stroke; adverse pregnancy outcomes	Smoked or oral
Opiates (narcotics)				
Codeine	Various combinations with other drugs (e.g., Tylenol-3, Robitussin A-C)	Captain Cody, cody, schoolboy, cods, deens, fours	*Common to opiates:* Pain relief, euphoria, drowsiness / *Common to opiates:* Nausea, constipation, confusion, sedation; respiratory depression and arrest; unconsciousness, coma, death	Oral and injected
Morphine	Roxanol, Duramorph	M, Miss Emma, Aunt Emma, monkey, white silk, white stuff		Oral, injected, and smoked
Opium	N/A	Big O, black stuff, block, gum, hop		Oral and smoked
Heroin	N/A	Brown sugar, dope, H, horse, junk, skag, skunk, smack, white horse, 8, A-bomb, Aunt Hazel, Big Daddy		Smoked, snorted, and injected
Oxycodone hydrochloride	OxyContin	Oxy, O.C., killer		Oral, snorted, and injected
Hydrocodone bitartrate with acetaminophen	Vicodin	Vike, Waston-387		Oral
Fentanyl	Actiq, Duragesic, Sublimaze	Apache, China girl, China white, dance fever, friend, goodfella, jackpot, murder 8, TNT, Tango and Cash, fen		Injected, smoked, and snorted

(continued)

TABLE 3.1. (continued)

Drug name	Commercial names	Common street names (slang)	Potential intoxication effects	Potential negative effects	Routes of administration
Club drugs					
Lysergic acid diethylamide (LSD)	N/A	Acid, blotter, boomers, caps, cubes, dots, microdot, sunshine pills	Altered states of perception and feeling; euphoria	Increased body temperature, heart rate, and blood pressure; loss of appetite; sleeplessness, numbness, weakness, tremors, flashbacks	Oral (absorbed through tissues of the mouth)
Methylenedioxyme-thamphetamine (MDMA)	N/A	Adam, clarity, Ecstasy, Eve, lover's speed, peace, STP, X, XTC	Mild hallucinogenic effects; increased tactile sensitivity; empathic feelings; euphoria, general stimulation	Problems with learning and memory; hyperthermia, cardiac toxicity, renal failure, liver toxicity; reduced appetite, weight loss; insomnia, nervousness	Oral
Cannabis					
Marijuana	N/A	Dope, ganja, grass, herb, joint, Mary Jane, pot, reefer, smoke, stash, rope, weed	*Common to cannabis:* Euphoria, slowed thinking, decreased reaction time	*Common to cannabis:* Confusion; problems with balance and coordination; frequent coughs or respiratory infections; impaired learning and memory; anxiety; panic attacks, increased heart rate	Smoked or oral
Hashish	N/A	Boom, chronic, gangster, hash, hemp			
Inhalants					
Solvents (e.g., paint thinners, gasoline, glues)	Various brand names	N/A	*Common to inhalants:* Euphoria, general stimulation, loss of inhibition	*Common to inhalants:* Headache, nausea, vomiting; problems with speech and motor coordination; wheezing, unconsciousness, cramps, weight loss, muscle weakness, depression, memory impairment; damage to cardiovascular and nervous systems; sudden death	Inhaled through mouth or nose
Gases (e.g., butane, propane, aerosol propellants, nitrous oxide)	Various brand names	N/A			
Nitrites (e.g., isoamyl, isobutyl, cyclohexyl)	Various brand names	Laughing gas, poppers, snappers, whippets			

Note. Information in this table is based on the following sources: Abadinsky (2004); Hansen and Venturelli (2001); NIDA (2003); Pagliaro and Pagliaro (1996).

person's *blood alcohol concentration* (BAC). As this name suggests, the BAC refers to the amount of alcohol the person has in the bloodstream. The BAC depends on a number of factors, including the amount a person is drinking; the concentration of alcohol in the drink (e.g., "hard liquors" such as gin or rum have higher alcohol concentration levels than beer); the presence or absence of food in the stomach; and the person's body composition as indicated by the fat-to-muscle ratio (Hanson & Venturelli, 2001). In general, people will experience more negative effects of alcohol if they have not eaten, are consuming many drinks with a high alcohol concentration in a short period of time, and have a higher fat-to-muscle ratio. In most states, a person is considered to be driving under the influence of alcohol when his or her BAC measures between 0.08% and 0.10% (National Institute on Alcohol Abuse and Alcoholism [NIAAA], 2001).

Barbiturates

Barbiturates are used in medical settings for such purposes as controlling pain, producing sedation, reducing anxiety, and inducing sleep (Abadinsky, 2004; NIDA, 2005). However, barbiturates constitute a very dangerous class of depressants, because there is a high risk of coma and death from overdose (especially when they are combined with other drugs, such as other pain relievers or alcohol). As with other depressants, there is also a high risk of developing tolerance to barbiturates, and serious medical complications such as seizures, coma, and death can result when people are withdrawing from these substances.

Benzodiazepines

Benzodiazepines are widely prescribed to reduce anxiety as well as to produce sedation and sleep (Abadinsky, 2004; NIDA, 2005f). Benzodiazepines are commonly referred to as "minor tranquilizers," because they produce many of the same effects of barbiturates but pose lower risks of death from overdose and withdrawal. The risk of developing tolerance to benzodiazepines is also generally lower than that for barbiturates; however, the same medical cautions described for barbiturates above also apply to benzodiazepines.

Other Depressants

We want to mention three additional depressants because of their high propensity for abuse. Rohypnol (flunitrazepam) more commonly known as "rophies" or the "date rape drug," is technically a benzodiazepine and has similar effects (e.g., sedation and drowsiness); however, it also produces a period of memory loss that coincides with the time a person is under the influence of the drug (National Institute on Drug Abuse [NIDA], 2006). Many stories in the popular media involve this drug being slipped into someone's drink without that person's knowledge and then producing blackouts for subsequent events. Similarly, gamma-hydroxybutyrate (GHB) is a depressant that produces the effects of drowsiness and sleep, and at high doses can produce loss of consciousness and death (NIDA, 2006). GHB is another drug that has been used to render a potential victim unconscious in relation to sexual assaults. Finally, methaqualone (e.g., Quaalude) is a depressant that produces barbiturate-like effects but also causes loss of bodily coordination (Abadinsky, 2004). In addition, persons taking methaqualone can quickly develop tolerance, and this drug has potentially lethal consequences from overdose and withdrawal. So far, we have discussed drugs that depress bodily functions; we now turn to substances that stimulate the CNS.

Stimulants

As the name suggests, *stimulants* speed up the CNS. In general, stimulants are used to increase energy level and mental alertness, as well as to fend off feelings of being tired or sleepy. In addition, these drugs are associated with physiological increases in blood pressure, respiration, and heart rate. One of the most commonly used stimulants is caffeine, which can be found in coffee, tea, and soda. Nicotine is another commonly used and highly addictive stimulant and is found in cigarettes, cigars, and chewing tobacco. The use of nicotine via cigarettes and chewing tobacco is linked to the adverse and potentially fatal consequences of lung and mouth cancer. There are many other types of stimulants, and many of these also have abuse potential.

Amphetamines

Amphetamines are very potent drugs that are used to produce an exaggerated sense of well-being (euphoria), as well as highly increased energy levels. Methamphetamine has become one of the most commonly abused drugs in this category in the United States. Methamphetamine is made cheaply and typically sold illegally in the form of a white powder, which is commonly smoked. The manufacturing of methamphetamine is a very dangerous process, as many highly volatile and toxic chemicals are used; thus law enforcement officials generally take special safety precautions when busting a "meth lab." Methamphetamine is frequently abused because it is relatively cheap to buy (compared to cocaine) and produces a rapid high that can last from 5 to 30 minutes (Abadinsky, 2004). Because appetite suppression is another common effect of methamphetamine, it allows individuals to control their weight more easily than via conventional methods such as exercise and good eating habits. Long-term use of this drug damages cells in the brain that regulate neurotransmitters such as dopamine, and it can produce parkinsonian movement disorders (NIDA, 2005e).

Cocaine

Cocaine produces a rapid increase in energy level, mental alertness, and general sense of well-being. This drug typically comes in the form of a white powder, which is snorted via the nose or injected in a vein after being dissolved in water. The physiological effects of cocaine include constricted blood vessels, as well as increased body temperature, heart rate, and blood pressure (NIDA, 2005b). The high from snorting cocaine is not long-lasting and generally ranges from 15 to 30 minutes. As a rule, cocaine is expensive to buy, but a cheaper street version known as "crack" can be smoked and produces a rapid though even briefer high (lasting between 5 and 10 minutes). Due to the relatively short duration of these highs, it is not uncommon for individuals to increase their cocaine dosage in order to extend the euphoric feelings it produces.

Ritalin

Although Ritalin (methylphenidate) is a commonly prescribed drug for students with attention-deficit/hyperactivity disorder (ADHD), it is included here because it has also been abused by students in school settings. It does not appear that individuals with ADHD are themselves at risk for abusing this drug when it is taken as prescribed (Abadinsky, 2004; NIDA, 2005f); however, some students who have been prescribed Ritalin for ADHD may sell it to other students. The individuals most at risk for abusing Ritalin are those who do not have ADHD but take the drug in order to experience its stimulating effects, such as increased energy, heightened alertness, and decreased fatigue. In addition, the physiological effects of this drug are similar to those of other stimulants.

Opioids

Opioids (also commonly referred to as *narcotics*) take their name from the opium poppy, which people have known for centuries has medicinal value. In medical settings, opioids are used because of their analgesic properties; that is, they are employed to manage pain. In particular, opioids are used to reduce the pain associated with surgery and other medical procedures, as well as to treat chronic pain conditions. These drugs are abused because of their ability to produce euphoria and a feeling of drowsiness, which are associated with their analgesic properties. The physiological effects of these drugs include constipation and respiratory depression; opioids can be fatal if taken in large doses because of their effects on respiration. In general, it is not safe to mix these drugs with depressants such as alcohol, barbiturates, or benzodiazepines, because these drugs also decrease respiration, and the combined effect can easily be lethal. The consistent use of opioids can lead to tolerance, and withdrawal from these drugs should be monitored by a medical professional. In addition, medications such as methadone, buprenorphine, and naltrexone are commonly used to treat the symptoms of opioid withdrawal. For the sake of simplicity, we have categorized opioids into two general categories: (1) codeine, morphine, and heroin; and (2) prescription medications containing other opioids.

Codeine, Morphine, and Heroin

If you have undergone any type of minor surgery, you may have been prescribed a pain reliever that contained either codeine or morphine to manage pain associated with the procedure; codeine is also commonly found in prescription cough syrup, as it is a cough suppressant (NIDA, 2005f). Thus many students may gain access to these drugs by looking through their parents' medicine cabinets. Codeine and morphine are abused by students in order to experience euphoria and general feelings of relaxation. However, both of these drugs also carry high risks of creating tolerance, as well as of severe withdrawal symptoms after a period of consistent use.

Heroin is a derivative of morphine. It is typically sold in the form of a white or brown powder, which can be injected intravenously, snorted, or smoked. People use heroin in order to experience a euphoric state commonly referred to as a "rush." This rush is generally associated with dry mouth, warm flushing sensation of the skin, and feelings of heaviness in the hands and feet (NIDA, 2005c). Typically following the rush is a period of up to 2 hours in which the person experiences alternating wakeful and drowsy states. Mental functioning is generally impaired during the post-rush period, due to heroin's depressive effects on the CNS. Long-term heroin use produces severe negative consequences, including heart infections, collapsed veins, abscesses, and liver disease; intravenous use also creates an increased risk for infectious diseases such as HIV and hepatitis. In general, heroin users quickly develop tolerance for the drug, and long-term users can experience withdrawal symptoms within a few hours after using the drug. The withdrawal symptoms of heroin have been described as resembling severe flu symptoms; they include insomnia, restlessness, intense craving for the drug, severe body pain, diarrhea and vomiting, sweats, cold flashes, and involuntary kicking movements. In addition, heroin can cause death when used in large doses, as it severely depresses the CNS.

Prescription Medications Containing Other Opioids

Professionals working in school settings have probably heard of students abusing prescription medications such as OxyContin and Vicodin. These medications contain opioids that are chemically similar but not identical to codeine. In medical settings, these drugs are prescribed to patients for their pain-relieving properties, and again students can probably access them by looking through their parents' medicine cabinets. Individuals abuse these medications to experience the euphoria and sedated state associated with the pain-relieving properties of these drugs. These medications generally carry the same negative consequences and risks (e.g., death from overdose) as other opioid-based drugs (NIDA, 2005f). In addition, these drugs should not be combined with depressants such as alcohol or barbiturates, because both classes of substances depress the CNS and can cause death when mixed.

Club Drugs

The so-called "club drugs" are substances that are typically used in nightclub settings and at young adult parties called "raves" where drug use is the norm. The drugs in this category include but are not limited to lysergic acid diethylamide (LSD), methylenedioxymethamphetamine (MDMA or Ecstasy), mushrooms, GHB, Rohypnol, and ketamine.

Although some of these drugs technically fall into other categories (e.g., Rohypnol and GHB are depressants, as described above), we include them in this category because of their association with clubs and parties. Individuals take these drugs to experience euphoria and the distorted perceptions of reality produced by heightened sensations of sight and sound. It should be noted that the individual drugs' effects may vary. For example, LSD is a hallucinogenic drug that severely distorts the perception of reality by stimulating the CNS and disrupting its ability to regulate information from the senses (Abadinsky, 2004). Individuals who take LSD typically experience hallucinations, illusions, and a heightened sense of reality, but these effects are dependent on the amount used. Other effects of LSD include rapid mood swings, experiencing several feelings at once, and delusions (NIDA, 2005d), The effects of LSD generally occur 30–90 minutes after consumption and can last up to 12 hours; experiencing the effects of LSD over a period of hours is termed a "trip." The physiological effects of LSD include increases in body temperature, heart rate, and blood pressure, as well as sweating, appetite loss, insomnia, dilated pupils, dry mouth, and tremors. Some individuals who use LSD experience "flashbacks," which occur in the days, weeks, or months following use. A flashback is a spontaneous experience of components of the original drug-induced episode.

MDMA or Ecstasy is another club drug that technically belongs in the stimulant category and produces both stimulant and hallucinogenic effects. For example, MDMA users generally experience increases in energy, a sense of euphoria, and mild illusions and hallucinations. Taking large doses of this drug affects the body's ability to regulate temperature and can cause a condition called *hyperthermia*, which results in failure of the kidneys, liver, and cardiovascular system and can lead to death (NIDA, 2005a). When this drug is used at a party, an adolescent user could be dancing for hours before noticing that he or she is dehydrated or feeling a significant increase in body temperature. Long-term MDMA use is associated with deficits in learning and memory, as well as with depressive symptoms many days after the drug was actually used. Individuals who use LSD and MDMA can develop tolerance for them, but generally not withdrawal symptoms.

Marijuana

Marijuana is the illicit substance most commonly abused by adolescents. It comes from the hemp plant *Cannabis sativa* and is sold in the form of dried green or brown leaves. A highly concentrated form of this drug is termed *hashish*. Marijuana contains the chemical delta-9-tetrahydrocannabinol (THC), which produces the euphoric effects of the substance by connecting itself to cannabinoid receptors in the brain (NIDA, 2004b). Individuals typically smoke marijuana to experience euphoria and a sense of relaxation (which includes slowed thinking and responses, but can also include a general feeling of disorientation or confusion). Common negative physiological effects of regular marijuana use include frequent coughs and respiratory infections; negative psychological effects include lowered inhibitions and motivation (Abadinsky, 2004). Negative effects of long-term marijuana use include problems with learning, memory, concentration, problem solving, perception, and coordination, as well as increased heart rate. Marijuana smoke contains 50–70% more carcinogens than tobacco smoke and thus increases a person's chances of developing respiratory problems and lung cancer (Hoffmann, Brunneman, Gori, & Wynder, 1975; Sridhar et al., 1994). Users can easily develop a tolerance to marijuana, but it is one of the few drugs that does not seem to produce physical withdrawal symptoms. However, it can produce psychological withdrawal symptoms, including an intense craving that is only lessened after the drug is used again.

Inhalants

Inhalants comprise over 1,000 products that can be inhaled through the nose and mouth and are commonly found in households. Inhalants produce a rapid and short-lasting high that includes the effects of stimulation, loss of inhibition, and anesthesia (i.e., a slowing down of bodily functions). Inhalant users typically take repeated doses or "hits" of a substance in order to extend the short-lived high. Repeated use of some inhalants such as butane, propane, and aerosol sprays can induce a condition called *sudden sniffing death*, which results from heart failure (NIDA, 2004a). The immediate negative effects of inhalant use include headaches, nausea and vomiting, problems with speech (e.g., slurred speech), and problems with body movement (e.g., poor motor coordination). Long-term effects include severe and sometimes irreversible damage to the CNS, as well as damage to hearing and bone marrow (NIDA, 2004a); in addition, damage to the liver and kidneys is possible.

National statistics indicate that inhalant use is more prevalent among 8th-grade students than among students in either 10th or 12th grade (Johnston, O'Malley, Bachman, & Schulenberg, 2005). This is probably the case because younger adolescents can easily access many inhalants in their homes and because the expense is much lower than for other drugs (such as alcohol and marijuana). Inhalants include a wide variety of individual substances, but are generally categorized into the following three categories: volatile solvents, gases, and nitrites (NIDA, 2004a).

The category containing the largest number of inhalants is volatile solvents (Hanson & Venturelli, 2001). A *solvent* is a substance that dissolves another substance; *volatile* refers to the capacity for part of a substance to evaporate quickly when exposed to the air. For example, nail polish remover is a volatile solvent because it dissolves nail polish on fingernails and because part of it evaporates quickly when exposed to the air. If you have used nail polish remover yourself or have been around someone using it, you have probably noticed a pungent odor associated with this substance. To take this example a step further, you may have also experienced a mild headache or feelings of nausea if you were in close proximity to the nail polish remover (or using it in a poorly ventilated area) for even a brief period of time. If so, you have experienced the general effects of using a volatile solvent. Other common volatile solvents include such things as paint thinner and paint removers, fluids used for dry cleaning, other cleaning chemicals (e.g., degreasers, spot removers), gasoline, and glue.

Typical *gases* used as inhalants include butane, propane, the aerosol dispensers used in whipped cream bottles ("whippets"), hair sprays, and spray paints. The category of inhalants called *nitrites* is less commonly abused (due to more limited availability) than the other inhalants. Nitrites, also referred to as *poppers,* cause vasodilatation (the opening of blood vessels) in the body and are sometimes used medically to treat severe angina pectoris (Hanson & Venturelli, 2001). These substances were made illegal to sell in the United States during the early 1990s; however, they can be purchased over the Internet from other countries and are found in some adult stores. They are typically packaged in small brown bottles labeled as containing other products, such as liquid aroma, room deodorizer, leather cleaner, or video head cleaner (NIDA, 2004a).

As you can see from the preceding discussion, there are many substances of abuse. The euphoric effects of each substance and the medical risks of taking it vary, depending on how the specific substance interacts with the CNS. In general, these substances initially produce euphoria or a high that the user experiences as pleasurable. Continued use of a substance typically produces symptoms of tolerance and withdrawal, and the speed at which these symptoms develop will also depend on the specific substance abused. Again, Table 3.1 can serve as a quick reference for information on drugs of abuse. Now that we have provided information on what types of drugs are abused, their effects on the body, and the risks of taking them, we focus on the process of screening students for substance abuse.

SCREENING FOR A SUBSTANCE ABUSE PROBLEM

It has been our experience that many school mental health professionals do not feel as if they have the necessary information or training to screen or assess students for a substance abuse problem, although they believe that such information and training are important to obtain because of the problems they see students having with drugs. In fact, results from two recent national survey studies of high school and middle school counselors indicated that screening and assessment were rated as the most important areas in which to receive substance-abuse-related training (Burrow-Sanchez & Lopez, in press; Burrow-Sanchez, Lopez, & Slagle, in press). These results are not surprising, given the two questions we are most commonly asked by school personnel: "How do I know if a student is abusing substances?" and "If a student has a problem with substances, how do I know how severe it is?" We realize that most schools do not have substance abuse specialists on staff or the resources necessary to provide comprehensive assessment. Therefore, our primary focus in this section of the chapter is on brief screening methods that can be easily implemented by school mental health professionals with minimal prior training in substance abuse. An important caveat is that school professionals will need to follow all school, district, and state policies and statutes for obtaining student and parental consent to screen or assess for a substance abuse problem. We discuss consent and confidentiality issues next (see Chapter 1 for more information).

Issues of Consent and Confidentiality

Before any type of screening for a substance abuse problem takes place, school mental health professionals will need to address relevant issues of consent and confidentiality. We assume that all such professionals are familiar with the policies and practices for obtaining parental consent and student assent in their schools. It is also important to realize that information related to substance abuse is protected by federal regulations (42 CFR; see Chapter 1 for a discussion).

Some schools may require parental consent to be obtained before a school mental health professional has any discussion with a student about potential substance abuse, while other schools may permit one meeting with a student before parental consent must be obtained. Parents usually provide *consent* for their son or daughter, whereas the student provides his or her *assent* or *agreement* due to being a minor. Some exceptions to these guidelines are made if the student is age 18 (a legal adult) or is legally emancipated from his or her parents. It is also important to note that states have varying laws about the age at which a minor can consent to certain types of medical treatment (including substance abuse treatment) without the consent of his or her parents. In fact, the American Bar Association has produced a downloadable booklet titled *Facts about Children and the Law* (see *www.abanet.org*), which provides an overview of states' laws on this issue. However, we strongly recommend that you check with officials in your own state regarding the age at which minors can consent to medical treatment without the consent of their parents, and the types of treatment that are included.

Confidentiality is another issue that must be addressed early in the screening process. In practice, it is best if the school mental health professional, the student, and his or her parents all agree about how confidentiality will be handled. Again, schools and districts may have specific procedures, guidelines, or laws related to the confidentiality of substance abuse information; also, again, 42 CFR specifically addresses the confidentiality of information related to substance abuse. We believe that as a school mental health professional, you should address issues of confidentiality at the same time you obtain parental consent and student assent. In particular, you should specifically indicate what types of information will be shared with whom and for what purposes. For example, a mother may want to know everything her son discloses to you, including his level of drug use. The student may fear that his mother will be told whatever he discloses to you, including information about his drug use. Such a situation can quickly place you in an uncomfortable predicament. However, we suggest that you make it clear just what types of information will be shared with a student and his or her parents, and provide the reasons for doing (or not doing) so. This could include your informing the parents that the student is likely to disclose little information about a potential substance abuse problem if he or she fears that anything said will also be reported to a parent. In short, we recommend being as clear as possible with students and parents regarding issues of confidentiality, in keeping with any relevant local or national professional guidelines, policies, or laws on this matter. Once issues of consent and confidentiality have been addressed, screening for substance abuse can move forward.

Defining Screening and Assessment for a Substance Problem

Screening

Screening for potential substance abuse can be conducted by a school mental health professional and can provide valuable information to assist the student, parents, and school in dealing with a potential problem. The goal of screening is to quickly provide enough information to indicate whether a more thorough assessment is needed. For example, suppose a student is caught with marijuana in his or her locker. Based on this limited amount of information, it is difficult to know how much at risk this particular student is for substance abuse. When questioned, the student can respond in a variety of ways, such as "It's not mine; I was holding it for someone else!" or "Yes, it's mine, but I haven't even tried it yet!" On the surface, these types of responses are not very helpful to the school professional who is trying to understand the problem.

We realize that in some schools, screening students for a substance abuse problem may be in direct conflict with established zero tolerance policies as described in Chapter 1. In schools that have graduated systems of consequences for student problem behaviors, such as early response (again, see Chapter 1), school mental health professionals may have more latitude in working with students. Therefore, the readers of this book need to determine in what ways the screening-related information we discuss in this chapter is relevant to their particular school settings. We discuss the specifics of screening below, but we first provide a brief description of comprehensive assessment procedures, in order to familiarize school mental health professionals with the general assessment process (even though most of this chapter focuses on screening). We refer the reader to Chapter 5 for more specific information on comprehensive assessment within the context of providing individual interventions for substance abuse.

Assessment

The main goal of a comprehensive assessment is to gain a full and accurate understanding of a student's substance abuse, once the likelihood of a substance problem has been identified through screening. Specifically, information from such an assessment will assist a school mental health professional in determining how severe the problem is and what type of intervention will be most appropriate. A comprehensive substance abuse assessment typically includes the following components: a semistructured clinical interview with the adolescent by a trained professional; collection of information from others close to the adolescent (e.g., parents, school personnel); and administration of standardized self-report measures on drug use and other problem behaviors. Some schools may also require an adolescent to submit to urinalysis as part of the assessment. The information gathered during the assessment process should culminate with a determination of the most appropriate type of intervention, depending on the severity of the problem, the presence of any co-occurring disorders, and other characteristics of the adolescent and family. If comprehensive assessment services are not available for students in some schools, then referrals to appropriate community agencies are warranted. Regardless of the screening or assessment methods used, however, there needs to be a positive working relationship between the school mental health professional and the student in order for valid results to be obtained.

Establishing a Positive Working Relationship

Among the potential difficulties in working with students who may have substance problems are their reluctance to talk openly about the issue and their tendency to underreport drug use (Winters, Stinchfield, Henly, & Schwartz, 1992). In many school settings, student substance problems fall under the zero tolerance policies, and students are punished for any and all drug-related behaviors. In the community, adolescents with substance abuse problems are most often referred to treatment centers by juvenile justice courts, schools, or parents (Muck et al., 2001). Therefore, by the time a student reaches a school mental health professional for substance abuse screening, he or she may already have been in trouble with someone else (e.g., school administration, parents, juvenile justice authorities) regarding the issue.

Most students are keenly aware that disclosure of substance use is likely to lead to serious negative consequences rather than support. Students may also anticipate that adults in positions of authority (such as school mental health professionals) will tell them such things as "You must stop using drugs immediately" and "This is a bad thing you are doing." Therefore, it is not unreasonable for students with substance abuse problems to approach adults in school settings with a high degree of resistance.

Working *with* an adolescent's resistance (not against it) is one of the most important first steps in developing a positive working relationship with the student (Miller & Rollnick, 2002). Building a sense of trust and understanding early in the relationship will help to reduce the student's resistance to talking about his or her substance use. One particular strategy is to initiate a discussion with the student about what will be done with the information discussed. Most students will be apprehensive about discussing their drug use history for fear that their information will be shared with parents, school administrators, or legal authorities, and that negative consequences will ensue. Initiating a discussion about how drug-use-related information will and will not be used, along with who will and will not have access to it, can go a long way toward lowering the students' resistance to talking with a school mental health professional. Thus we recommend being frank with students regarding what policies and procedures on substance use exist in their schools and how these things affect the information students share.

A second strategy to lower resistance is to listen for challenges an adolescent is currently facing (e.g., disciplinary consequences at school, problems at home) and use the skills of reflection to echo his or her statements back in a way that communicates an understanding of the student's situation (Miller & Rollnick, 2002). To illustrate this strategy, we present the following two scenarios between a high school student and a school counselor:

Scenario 1

HIGH SCHOOL STUDENT: My parents have really been getting on to me about using marijuana. They said they won't let me drive the car any more if I don't stop using!

SCHOOL COUNSELOR: I don't blame your parents! Why are you using marijuana? You should stop using that stuff; don't you know how bad it is for you?

HIGH SCHOOL STUDENT: You sound just like my parents! I knew it would be a waste of time to talk to you about this!

SCHOOL COUNSELOR: Well, all you need to do is stop using marijuana, and your problems will be solved!

Scenario 2

HIGH SCHOOL STUDENT: My parents have really been getting on to me about using marijuana. They said they won't let me drive the car any more if I don't stop using!

SCHOOL COUNSELOR: Sounds like your marijuana use is causing problems for you at home with your parents, and you are worried about losing some important privileges, like driving. Is that right?

HIGH SCHOOL STUDENT: Yeah, that's right, and I'm not sure what to do about it.

SCHOOL COUNSELOR: Would it be helpful to brainstorm ways that you can work on your problems at home with your parents?

HIGH SCHOOL STUDENT: Yeah, I think that would be good!

In the first scenario, the school counselor says things that many of us believe about adolescent substance use (in effect, "Don't use drugs and you won't have any problems!"), but that are not particularly helpful in establishing a positive working relationship with the student. Generally, direct confrontation about not using substances will shut down the lines of communication between a school mental health professional and a student. In the second scenario, the counselor does not directly address the student's substance use, but rather places it within the context of the student's current problems. At the same time, the counselor keeps the student engaged in a conversation as opposed to limiting it, which is what occurs in the first scenario. The counselor in the second scenario will probably be able to continue having a constructive discussion with the student about ways to solve his or her problems. In doing so, the counselor is also beginning to establish a positive working relationship with the student. The establishment of such a relationship will allow the counselor to probe the student about his or her substance use more directly and with less resistance. These two scenarios illustrate how a school mental health school professional can either engage or disengage a student very quickly within the first few sentences of a conversation. The use of this reflection technique allows the student to feel heard by the school mental health professional and will facilitate the establishment of a positive working relationship.

In general, adolescents will respond better to discussing a sensitive topic such as substance use when they perceive the environment to be supportive and nonthreatening, and when the emphasis is on understanding the problem instead of placing blame on them (Baer & Peterson, 2002). Lowering a student's resistance as described above will allow him or her to communicate more openly about a possible substance problem and will help the school mental health professional to gather more accurate information. Many other useful suggestions for working individually with students are included in Chapter 5.

STEPS IN THE SCREENING PROCESS

We have developed the Student Screening Decision Sheet (SSDS; see Figure 3.1) in order to provide school mental health professionals with guidelines for screening students for potential substance abuse problems. The SSDS lists four major steps for a professional to work through with a student in a sequential manner. We now discuss each of these steps in turn.

Step 1: Is Screening Necessary?

In the first step of the SSDS, a school mental health professional should determine whether screening for substance abuse is necessary for the student in question. We suggest that if the professional is even considering this question, the answer will almost always be "yes." In school settings, this question typically arises in response to specific circumstances concerning a student. We define these specific circumstances more generally in Figure 3.1 as "Risk Category A: Direct information about substance-use-related problems at school" and "Risk Category B: Multiple risk factors present." The school professional should consider whether the student's behavior and related information fit into one of these categories.

Risk Category A covers instances in which a school mental health professional has prior knowledge of a potential substance abuse problem before discussing it with the student. School professionals typically obtain this type of information in the following ways: (1) A student is caught in possession of drugs at school; (2) the student comes to school under the influence of drugs; or (3) another person, such as a teacher, parent, or peer, provides information about suspicion of drug use. Any of these events constitutes a good reason for the school professional to conduct a screening with the student.

Risk Category B covers instances in which a student exhibits multiple risk factors for substance abuse (see Chapter 2 for a review of risk factors). In general, the presence of a single risk factor by itself does not indicate that a student is experiencing a problem with substances. For example, low academic achievement is a risk factor for substance abuse, but on its own does not indicate that a substance problem exists. (An exception to this general rule is that certain risk factors, such as peer use of substances, are more highly related to adolescent substance use than others.) Therefore, a school mental health pro-

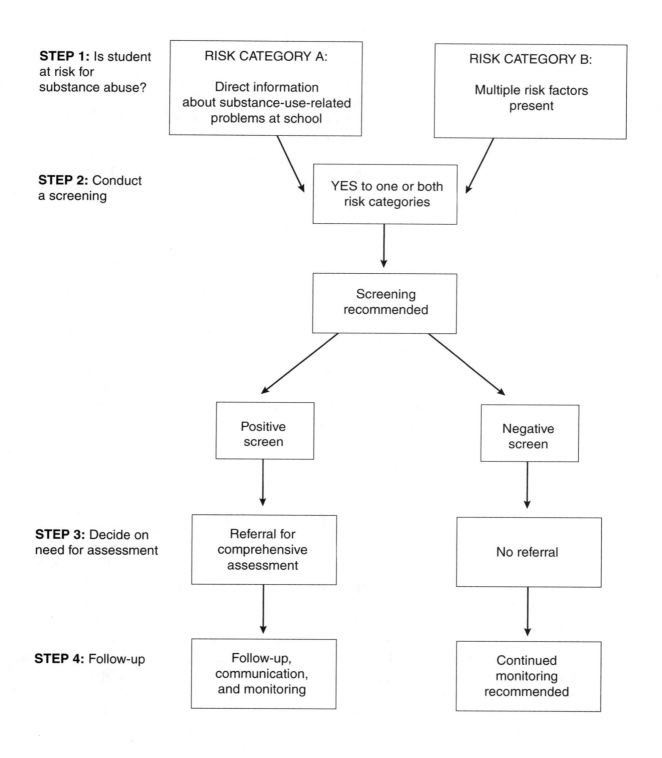

STEP 1: Is student at risk for substance abuse?

RISK CATEGORY A:

Direct information about substance-use-related problems at school

RISK CATEGORY B:

Multiple risk factors present

STEP 2: Conduct a screening

YES to one or both risk categories

Screening recommended

Positive screen

Negative screen

STEP 3: Decide on need for assessment

Referral for comprehensive assessment

No referral

STEP 4: Follow-up

Follow-up, communication, and monitoring

Continued monitoring recommended

FIGURE 3.1. Student Screening Decision Sheet (SSDS).

fessional should usually be more concerned with the presence of multiple risk factors for a student.

Newcomb (1995) found a positive relationship between the number of risk factors present and the frequency of drug use for adolescents. In other words, as adolescents were exposed to more risk factors, their use of drugs also increased. The number of risk factors Newcomb examined ranged from none at the low end to five or more at the high end. As expected, adolescents who were exposed to five or more risk factors reported the most frequent drug use. Therefore, the presence of multiple risk factors is a strong indicator of potential substance abuse and of the need for screening.

Step 2: Conduct a Screening

Screening a student for substance abuse should be kept relatively brief, since the goal is to obtain enough information to decide whether a more comprehensive assessment is warranted. At a minimum, screening should consist of a brief interview with the student and administration of a self-report screening measure. The professional may also wish to obtain information from other people who know the student well, such as parents and teachers. If information is gathered from others, this should be done with the full awareness of the student, in order to promote trust and lower resistance in the working relationship. We discuss conducting a brief interview and administering a self-report measure next.

Brief Interview

Establishing a positive working relationship with the student as described above is absolutely essential to conducting a brief interview as part of the screening process. The main goal of this interview is to obtain information about the following areas: drug(s) the student is using; age at onset of drug use; frequency of drug use; and information about relevant risk factors, both intrapersonal (e.g., depressive symptoms) and interpersonal (e.g., family history of drug use). Clearly, it is important for the school mental health professional to identify the student's preferred drug of use, any other drugs that are part of the problem, and the frequency of use (e.g., daily, weekly, monthly). Establishing the student's age at onset of drug use is also important, because earlier initial use predicts more problems with substances at later ages (Anthony & Petronis, 1995; Hawkins, Catalano, & Miller, 1992). Finally, relevant intrapersonal and interpersonal risk factors for the student should be examined, in case any were overlooked in Step 1 of the SSDS (see also Table 2.1). In sum, gathering this type of information from the student will assist the school professional in obtaining a clearer picture of the actual drug problem.

A school mental health professional can include several additional areas of interest in the brief interview. First, the student can be asked about the reasons why he or she uses a particular substance (e.g., coping with stress, self-medication for depression), as well as about any negative consequences of drug use (e.g., problems with law enforcement, physical symptoms). Asking questions about these areas will help increase the student's awareness of a potential drug use problem without directly placing blame on the student for using substances. It is also important to screen for the presence of any co-occurring disorders, including but not limited to conduct disorder, ADHD, depression, anxiety disorders, and learning disorders (Riggs, 2003; Weinburg, 2001). Greenbaum, Foster-Johnson, and Petrila (1996) estimate that approximately 50% of adolescents who abuse substances have a co-occurring disorder. Asking about these additional areas will provide a fuller picture of a student's potential substance problem.

Screening Instruments

The school mental health professional can administer a self-report screening instrument to obtain more information about a student's potential substance abuse problem. Some students may be more comfortable answering questions on a paper-and-pencil measure than answering questions in an interview; thus school professionals may find it helpful to begin the screening process by administering a self-report measure and following it with a brief interview. Screening instruments are typically self-reports and range in length from fewer than 20 items to over 100. Some instruments are designed to focus on use of a specific drug (e.g., alcohol), whereas others cover a wider range of substance use and other potential problem areas (e.g., mental/physical health, family relationships). A listing of brief screening measures appropriate for use by school mental health professionals can be found in Table 3.2. We discuss two of these measures in more detail below.

The Adolescent Alcohol and Drug Involvement Scale (AADIS) is a 14-item screening instrument designed to measure both drug use history and the level of drug use (Moberg, 2000). The AADIS does not require any special training to administer and is in the public domain. This instrument takes approximately 5 minutes to administer and 2 minutes to score. The total scores obtained on the AADIS will assist the school mental health professional in determining whether a more comprehensive assessment is warranted for the student. A strength of the AADIS is that it can be administered and scored quickly, whereas a weakness is that it does not provide information about other potential problem areas (e.g., mental health, peers).

The Problem-Oriented Screening Instrument for Teenagers (POSIT) is a 139-item measure that was developed to screen for problems in 10 areas, including substance abuse, mental health, physical health, family relationships, and peer relations issues (Rahdert, 1991). The POSIT is designed to be used with adolescents ages 12–19 years and can be easily administered and scored by school mental health professionals. It can be administered to students either as a paper-and-pencil measure or on a computer. The administration time for the paper-and-pencil version is approximately 20–25 minutes, and it can be hand-scored in 2 minutes. In addition, English and Spanish versions of the instrument are available. The POSIT can be obtained through the National Clearinghouse for Alcohol and Drug Information (NCADI; see "Chapter Resources"). A strength of this measure is that it provides information about both substance use and other problem areas; a limitation is that it takes longer to administer than other screening instruments.

Making a decision about which instrument to select for screening purposes will depend on many factors: (1) type of information needed; (2) length/administration time; (3)

TABLE 3.2. Screening Measures

Screening measure	Length	Areas covered	Specialized training required?	Cost	Reference
Adolescent Alcohol Involvement Scale (AAIS)	14 items	Alcohol problems	No	Contact author	Mayer and Filstead (1979)
Adolescent Drinking Index (ADI)	24 items	Alcohol problems	Minimal training required	Yes—contact publisher (Psychological Assessment Resources)	Harrell and Wirtz (1989)
Adolescent Drug Involvement Scale (ADIS)	13 items	Drug problems other than alcohol	No	Public domain	Moberg and Hahn (1991)
Adolescent Alcohol and Drug Involvement Scale (AADIS)	14 items	Alcohol and other drug problems	No	Public domain	Moberg (2000)
Drug and Alcohol Problem Quick Screen (DAP)	30 items	Alcohol and other drug problems	No	Public domain	Schwartz and Wirtz (1990)
Personal Experience Screening Questionnaire (PESQ)	40 items	Alcohol and other drug problems	No	Yes—contact publisher (Western Psychological Services)	Winters (1992)
Problem-Oriented Screening Questionnaire for Teenagers (POSIT)	139 items	10 areas (Substance Abuse, Mental Health, etc.)	No	Public domain	Rahdert (1991)
Rutgers Alcohol Problem Index (RAPI)	23 items	Alcohol problems	No	Public domain	White and Labouvie (1989)

scoring procedures and ease of scoring; (4) type of prior training needed; (5) adequate psychometric properties, such as reliability and validity; (6) prior testing on groups of students similar to those in a particular school; and (7) cost. Once a suitable screening instrument is chosen, it can provide the school professional with additional information on which to base a decision about the need for a more comprehensive assessment.

Step 3: Decide on Need for Assessment

Using the information gathered during Step 2, the school mental health professional will make a decision regarding the need for further assessment. In some cases, the professional will easily be able to determine that further assessment is warranted for the student; we refer to this finding as a "positive screen" in the SSDS. In other cases, the data from Step 2 will indicate that further assessment is not warranted; we refer to this finding as a "negative screen" in the SSDS. Some schools may have the necessary resources for conducting a comprehensive assessment if one is needed, whereas others will not. In the latter case, the school professional will need to make an appropriate referral for the student to an agency in the community that can provide a proper assessment. As noted earlier, the results of this assessment should provide specific information on the severity of the student's substance abuse and the most appropriate type of intervention or treatment.

There will also be some cases in which the school mental health professional is unsure whether further assessment is needed, because the screening results do not appear conclusive. If you find yourself in this situation, we strongly suggest that you consult with another school professional or a professional in the community (assuming that confidentiality protections are in place), to discuss the results of the screening and obtain his or her opinion. Such a consultation is likely to assist you in clarifying whether an assessment is needed, and it may be particularly valuable if the screening results appear inconclusive but your clinical judgment or intuition indicates that the student should receive further assessment. For example, you may suspect that the student did not answer truthfully during the screening, and thus that the results are not valid. This is an excellent reason for consulting with an additional professional prior to making a decision regarding further assessment for the student.

Step 4: Follow-Up

In Step 3, you have decided that a comprehensive assessment is either warranted or not warranted for the student, based on the outcome of the screening. If your school has the resources to provide a comprehensive assessment for the student, then you can either conduct the assessment yourself (if you are qualified to do so) or follow up with the person at your school who conducts it. If, however, the student is referred for an assessment in the community, we suggest that you stay in contact with the agency, which is in the best interest of the student for a number of reasons. First, you can be a supportive resource for both the student and the agency as the assessment is conducted. Second, the results of the assessment will indicate the type of treatment needed, and you can assist in coordinating the student's academic needs with his or her treatment. Third, maintaining contact will probably indicate to the student and his or her family that you care about the outcome and will work with the student when he or she is integrated back into the school system. Finally, if a student does not receive further assessment (i.e., if the student's screen is negative), we still recommend that you continue to monitor the student informally for any additional signs of a potential substance problem. Some students who receive negative screens may still be appropriate for participation in school-based substance abuse prevention programs, such as psychoeducational groups.

CASE EXAMPLE

Tevita was a 16-year-old sophomore who had recently moved into a new school district and had been attending Nibley High School for about 3 months. Nibley School is situated on the north side of a large city and attracts families of middle to low socioeconomic status. His family had moved into the neighborhood from a very wealthy neighborhood on the south side, where Tevita had long-term, well-established friendships. His mother, recently divorced, was unable to afford housing in her old neighborhood and needed to move to be able to support Tevita and his younger brother.

One day Tevita's mother, Ms. Finau, called the school counselor, Spencer Carr, to discuss her concerns about Tevita. She shared with Spencer that her family was having a difficult time adjusting after the divorce and change in neighborhood. She had divorced her husband after many years of living with his alcoholism. Most recently, Mr. Finau had run head-on into another vehicle while driving drunk and had killed one of the passengers in the other vehicle. Tevita's brother had also been in the car and received significant injuries, which required extensive physical therapy. Ms. Finau was concerned that Tevita was depressed about the whole situation, and she suspected that he had started experimenting with drugs. She didn't like the kids he was hanging around with at his new school and thought they were a "bad influence" on him. She also reported that he was not completing his homework, and that several of his teachers had called her because he was refusing to do some in-class work. She asked the school counselor for some type of assessment related to substance abuse or depression.

Spencer gathered more information from Ms. Finau and agreed that given the number of risk factors and changes in Tevita's life, a substance abuse and mental health screening was warranted. He agreed to meet with Tevita to do a brief interview and administer a self-report measure. He asked Ms. Finau to talk with Tevita ahead of time, mention her concerns, and tell him that the school counselor would be meeting with him soon. Ms. Finau then signed the school district's consent form, which allowed Spencer to start the screening process.

During their initial meeting, Tevita was very unhappy about being called out of his favorite class to meet with Spencer. To try to create a more positive relationship, Spencer asked Tevita which time would be best to meet, and they agreed to meet during advisory period on Wednesday of that week. He mentioned to Tevita that the meetings might need to occur over more than one day, but that they could talk further about the best times and days to meet.

When Tevita met with Spencer on Wednesday, they discussed issues related to confidentiality and the school's policy toward drug use. Spencer shared that Tevita would not be suspended for any reported drug use, and he also described the types of information that would be shared with Ms. Finau. At first Tevita maintained that there were no problems and stated, "I am not sure why I'm here." Spencer replied that Tevita's mother had told him about a lot of changes in the family, which he guessed were pretty stressful for Tevita.

Spencer started the interview process by asking Tevita about his interests and his previous school experience. He also asked about his adjustment to the new school. During the meeting, Tevita became visibly upset (hands shaking, lips quivering) and disclosed that he had indeed been under a lot of stress at home and hated his new school. He missed his dad a lot and said that he only got to visit him in jail once every other week. He also shared that he was overwhelmed with having to care for his younger brother, including helping him shower and get to and from school.

Spencer asked what his new friends were like and what they liked to do for fun. Tevita mentioned that his friends often drank on weekends and disclosed that he too had tried alcohol. Spencer was particularly concerned when Tevita mentioned that he liked how alcohol "takes away the pain." Given the complex issues that Tevita presented, Spencer decided to administer the POSIT to provide a more comprehensive screening of potential problem areas. Tevita agreed to come back the following week to complete the POSIT.

Overall on the POSIT, Tevita scored at "high risk" in the following areas: substance abuse, mental health, and family relationships. He scored at "medium risk" in the area of aggressive behavior/delinquency. Based on these results, Spencer felt that Tevita was definitely in need of a more comprehensive assessment. He shared the information with Ms. Finau and asked whether she had insurance to cover this type of psychological evaluation. She stated that she had just started a new job and did not have medical coverage yet for the children. Spencer told her that a few low-cost community agencies had agreed to work with students from Nibley High School who needed mental health services beyond what the school could provide. He helped Ms. Finau schedule an appointment for a more comprehensive assessment, and mentioned that he would continue to meet with Tevita once a week to check in with him and see how he was doing. He also suggested that Tevita might benefit from participating in the psychoeducational substance prevention group, which was conducted by the school psychologist.

CHAPTER SUMMARY

One of the issues that school mental health professionals face is determining whether particular students are having problems with substances. In this chapter, we have focused on ways for school professionals to conduct brief screenings of students with suspected substance abuse problems. In order to conduct such screenings, school professionals should first have some understanding of the major drugs of abuse and their effects on the body, which we have described in the first section of the chapter. They should also be aware of consent/confidentiality issues, and should develop a reasonably good working relationship with any student they plan to screen. We have then described a four-step screening process for school professionals to follow: deciding whether screening is necessary; conducting the actual screening (which includes a brief interview with the student, as well as a screening instrument); deciding whether a comprehensive assessment is warranted; and following up with the student. Finally, a case example has illustrated how a school counselor implemented the screening process outlined in this chapter with a student at his school.

CHAPTER RESOURCES

National Institute on Drug Abuse (NIDA)
www.nida.nih.gov

This website has lots of great research-based information for students, parents, and school professionals regarding the major drugs of abuse and adolescent substance abuse. Much of this material is also available in Spanish.

NIDA for Teens

teens.drugabuse.gov/parents/index.asp

This is a website sponsored by NIDA and tailored specifically for adolescents.

National Institute on Alcohol Abuse and Alcoholism (NIAAA)

www.niaaa.nih.gov

This website has research-based information on the effects of alcohol, as well as on adolescent alcohol abuse. Two especially helpful publications are available through this site for a nominal cost:

- *Assessing Alcohol Problems: A Guide for Clinicians and Researchers* (Allen & Wilson, 2003). This research-based guide has a chapter specifically covering adolescent substance abuse assessment; it also provides coverage of the major screening and assessment measures used in the field as a whole.
- *Motivational Enhancement Therapy Manual* (Miller, Zweben, DiClemente, & Rychtarik, 1994). This manual was originally developed for treating adults with alcohol problems, but it (or components of it) can be adapted as needed for students.

National Clearinghouse for Alcohol and Drug Information (NCADI)

ncadi.samhsa.gov

This is a government-hosted website that provides thousands of resources on substance use and abuse, which can be directly ordered from the site. Most of the materials on this website can be obtained free of charge, including two particularly useful Treatment Improvement Protocol (TIP) publications from the Center for Substance Abuse Treatment (CSAT):

- *Enhancing Motivation for Change in Substance Abuse Treatment* (CSAT, 1999a). This publication includes information on the theoretical and practical aspects of motivational interviewing. It also contains many good forms and instruments related to the practice of motivational interviewing.
- *Screening and Assessing Adolescents for Substance Abuse Disorders* (CSAT, 1999b). This publication provides in-depth coverage of the screening and assessment process for adolescent substance abuse. It also provides coverage of the major instruments used for these purposes.

Alcohol and Drug Abuse Institute, University of Washington

lib.adai.washington.edu/instruments

This site provides a searchable database of almost 300 screening and assessment instruments related to substance abuse issues.

Motivational Interviewing

www.motivationalinterview.org

This is the official website for motivational interviewing and contains useful information, including where to obtain training, as well as comments from the developers.

4

Prevention Programming

Most school mental health professionals are familiar with the basic purposes of prevention programming, which are either to keep a potential problem from occurring or to keep an existing problem from becoming worse. Many programs are used in school settings to prevent such behaviors or conditions as disruptiveness, illiteracy, drug use, teenage pregnancy, and school dropout. The main goal of this chapter is to give school mental health professionals a better understanding of prevention strategies for student drug use and abuse. In order to accomplish this goal, we discuss the three levels of prevention programming, identify major principles of research-based prevention, provide in-depth examples of research-based programs, and present guidelines for implementing a school prevention program.

THE THREE LEVELS OF PREVENTION PROGRAMMING

Most school-based prevention programs are based on the idea that keeping a student from engaging in a potentially problematic behavior (e.g., substance use) is more beneficial to the student than trying to treat a problematic behavior after it has developed (e.g., substance abuse). In addition, research has found that *preventing* a behavior is more cost-effective than *treating* a behavior. For example, two studies indicate that for every $1 spent on prevention, approximately $4 to $10 is saved on substance abuse treatment (Pentz, 1998; Spoth, Guyull, & Day, 2002). This is a modern illustration of the old adage that "an ounce of prevention is worth a pound of cure." As most school mental health professionals know, many different school-based substance abuse prevention programs exist—but how do they decide which program is best for the types of students they work with or for their school setting? Just as there are many substance abuse prevention programs to choose from, there are also many factors to consider prior to choosing a program. We suggest beginning this process by answering this question: "At what level(s) does prevention programming need to occur in my school setting?"

A model for prevention that was originally developed in the public health arena and is appropriately applied here is the *three-tiered prevention model* (Mrazek & Haggerty, 1994). This model was originally developed by public health agencies as part of a larger intervention spectrum to address mental health disorders; it has also been adapted for use in school-based behavior intervention literature (see Walker et al., 1996). The three levels of this model are called *universal, selective,* and *indicated* prevention.

Figure 4.1 illustrates how this model fits within the context of schools. The *prevention triangle* depicted in this figure represents all of the students in a school and is divided into three levels. The level of prevention programming/support that students should receive is based on the severity of the problems presented by students. Specifically, a universal prevention program targets the entire student body through interventions that are implemented at the schoolwide level; that is, every student in the school receives such a program. One example of a universal prevention program for substance abuse is *LifeSkills Training* (LST; Botvin, 1998), which is reviewed later in this chapter. Research findings from school-based prevention programs for student problem behavior have indicated that the majority of students in a school will respond to universal prevention programming (Colvin, Kame'enui, & Sugai, 1993; Lewis & Sugai, 1999; Sugai, Horner, & Gresham, 2002). For a smaller percentage of students, selected prevention programs will be required. Selected prevention should target those students who are at risk for the development of a substance abuse or dependence disorder (Mrazek & Haggerty,

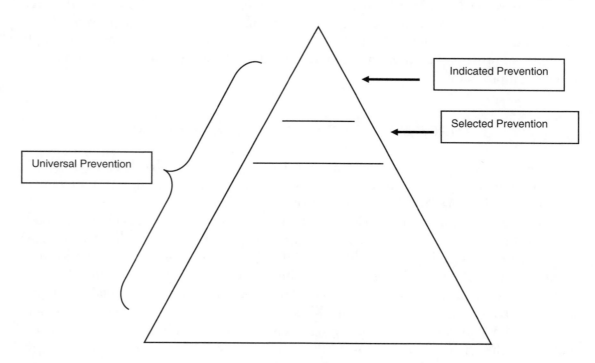

FIGURE 4.1. Prevention triangle.

1994). For example, a student who is caught with marijuana on campus or has a parent with a substance disorder is more likely than the average student to be at risk for developing a problem with substances. An example of a selected prevention program is the *Project Towards No Drug Abuse* (TND; Sussman, Dent, & Stacy, 2002), which is also described below.

The remaining student body will require even more intensive interventions. Indicated programs are the most intensive level of prevention and should target students who either show many signs or symptoms of substance abuse or dependence (see Mrazek & Haggerty, 1994) or meet the full mental health criteria for one of these disorders. Recent findings from the National Survey on Drug Use and Health (NSDUH) indicate that approximately 9% of youth between the ages of 12 and 17 meet mental health diagnostic criteria for a substance abuse or dependence disorder (Substance Abuse and Mental Health Services Administration [SAMHSA], 2006). These are the students who are most likely to have been referred to community mental health agencies for substance abuse assessment and treatment. These students will constitute only a small proportion of the entire student body; however, they will probably require more school personnel time because of their need for intensive school- and community-based interventions. An example of an indicated prevention program is Reconnecting Youth (RY; Eggert, Thompson, Herting, & Randall, 2001), which again is discussed more fully below.

As noted above, many school-based substance abuse prevention programs of all three types are available; some may be familiar to our readers, whereas others are unfamiliar. However, research has established that all effective prevention programs have certain principles in common. These principles are described next.

PRINCIPLES OF DRUG ABUSE PREVENTION

Recently the National Institute on Drug Abuse (NIDA) has published a guide for educators, community leaders, and parents that describes the major principles of substance abuse prevention programming (Robertson, David, & Rao, 2003). These principles, which have been derived from research on effective substance abuse prevention programs for youth, can be used in selecting, implementing, and evaluating such programs for children and adolescents. If you currently have a substance abuse prevention program in your school, determine how many of the principles below are included in your program. The following description of these principles is based on the NIDA publication (Robertson et al., 2003).

All substance abuse prevention programs for children and adolescents should:

1. Strengthen protective factors and concurrently decrease risk factors for youth.
2. Include information related to all types of drugs and drug abuse. Specifically, information on legal drugs (e.g., alcohol, cigarettes), illegal drugs (e.g., marijuana, cocaine), and other substances of abuse (e.g., inhalants, prescription medications) should be included.

3. Be tailored so that substance problems relevant to the local community are addressed.
4. Address the specific risks relevant to the characteristics (e.g., age, ethnicity, gender, socioeconomic status) of the local population.

Family-based substance abuse prevention programs should:

1. Include information and practice on:
   - Ways to strengthen family relationships (i.e., bonding).
   - Ways to enhance parenting skills.
   - Ways for families to develop and implement policies on substance abuse.
   - Inclusion of drug education information.

School-based substance abuse prevention programs should include specific information and practice at each school level:

1. The preschool level should focus on:
   - Improving prosocial behavior.
   - Improving social skills.
   - Building basic academic skills.
2. The elementary school level should focus on:
   - Improving academic skills (especially reading).
   - Improving social-emotional skills:
     - Self-control and emotional awareness.
     - Communication and problem solving.
3. The middle/junior and high school levels should focus on:
   - Improving academic and general social skills:
     - Study habits.
     - Communication.
     - Peer relationships.
     - Self-efficacy.
     - Assertiveness.
   - Building specific drug resistance skills.
   - Strengthening attitudes against drug use.
   - Strengthening personal commitments not to use drugs.
4. School-based programs should also include training for teachers on effective classroom behavior management, which can positively influence students' prosocial behavior, academic motivation/achievement, and school bonding.

Community-based programs should:

1. Target key developmental transitions for children and adolescents (e.g., the transition from elementary to middle school or from middle school to high school).
2. Combine two effective programs; for example, a combined school- and family-based program can be more effective than a school-based program alone.

3. Target multiple settings (e.g., schools, churches, clubs) in the community; however, these programs are most effective when they provide the same messages across settings.

When prevention programs are administered, they should:

1. Maintain the original research-based integrity of the program (i.e., its structure, content, and delivery) as much as possible, even when programs are adapted to meet local needs (e.g., local drug issues) and characteristics (e.g., cultural issues).
2. Be long term and include follow-up interventions such as booster sessions to strengthen the original goals of the program; for example, gains made by students from prevention programs in middle school will be reduced if not followed up in high school.
3. Employ interactive teaching strategies such as peer discussion groups and role playing, which serve to reinforce the information and skills being taught.

The above-described principles are helpful guidelines to assist school mental health professionals in deciding which substance abuse prevention program to implement, as well as in evaluating the current status of an existing program. However, these principles are still fairly general and do not provide specific descriptions of effective programs at each level of prevention. We have found that in addition to being aware of the principles, school professionals need to evaluate the specifics of each substance abuse prevention program being considered for implementation. Systematically evaluating several such programs in some detail will assist professionals in choosing the program that best meets the needs of students in their school setting. To help with the process of program selection, we provide a systematic way to evaluate research-based substance abuse prevention programs below, as well as descriptions of effective programs at the various levels of prevention.

EVALUATING RESEARCH-BASED PREVENTION PROGRAMS

School mental health professionals need to make many decisions prior to selecting a substance abuse prevention program for their school. As mentioned above, among the first questions that professionals should ask are "At what level(s) is substance abuse prevention programming needed in my school?" and "What are the specific needs of the students in my school?" Most prevention programs are designed to focus on one of the three specific levels of intervention—that is, universal, selected, or indicated. So this means that school professionals initially need to determine which level (or levels) is most appropriate for their school population at that particular time.

In selecting a specific program, school mental health professionals should also evaluate the core elements of prevention programs for relevancy in their setting. Robertson and colleagues (2003) describe the core elements of research-based programs as *structure*, *content*, and *delivery*. *Structure* refers to the program's prevention level (i.e., universal, selected, indicated); the target population (e.g., middle school students); and the setting in which the program will take place (e.g., school, community clinic). *Content* refers to the types of information that will be provided (e.g., drug education); the skills to be developed (e.g., problem-solving skills); the types of methods that will be used to support change (e.g., schoolwide rules); and the services to be delivered (e.g., school counseling, family therapy). *Delivery* refers to program selection and adaptation for particular populations (e.g., Hispanic adolescents), if required. It also refers to such aspects of implementation as program length and inclusion of booster sessions. Clearly, all of these core program elements are important for school mental health professionals to consider as they select among substance abuse prevention programs for their school. We next examine a program at each prevention level in terms of its core elements and the research evidence for its effectiveness, beginning with the universal level of prevention.

Evaluation of a Universal Prevention Program: LifeSkills Training

A universal substance abuse prevention program that has been studied extensively over the past several decades is the LifeSkills Training (LST) program (Botvin, 1998). LST is based on a competence enhancement model that is designed to improve general social and self-management skills for youth (Botvin, 2000). The major goal of LST is to teach youth not only relevant information, but also skills that will decrease the likelihood of their engaging in a range of problem behaviors, such as drug use and aggression. The three core skill sets taught in this program are drug resistance skills, personal self-management skills, and general social skills (LST, 2006). The program is designed to be delivered over a period of 3 academic years to middle school students. Students receive 15 program sessions in the first academic year, followed by 10 booster sessions in the second academic year. A final 5 sessions are delivered to students during the third academic year. The LST curriculum can be delivered by school personnel, such as teachers, school counselors, health educators, prevention specialists, and peer leaders; however, the program developers recommend that such personnel receive training in the LST curriculum prior to implementing it.

Research Support for LST

Botvin (2000) reported that findings from early research on LST indicated 40–80% reductions in the use of tobacco by students who had gone through the program compared to students who had not. He reported similar reductions in the use of alcohol and marijuana. Research evidence also suggests that the effects of LST do not wane considerably as these students continue to high school. For example, Botvin, Baker, Dusenbury, Botvin, and Diaz (1995) followed a large group of students through high school who had initially received the LST program in 7th grade, with additional sessions in 8th and 9th grades. These students were tracked and assessed at the end of 12th grade. Botvin and colleagues found that the use of alcohol, cigarettes, and marijuana was as much as 44%

lower for 12th-grade students who had received the LST intervention than for students who had not. In addition, research findings suggest that booster sessions are beneficial to maintain the preventive effects (Botvin, Renick, & Baker, 1983), and that the LST program is effective with Hispanic and African American youth (see Botvin, 2000). In sum, the LST program has strong research evidence to support its effectiveness in reducing drug use rates for students when implemented in middle school.

Core Elements of the LST Program

STRUCTURE

As noted above, LST is a universal prevention program, and the target group is middle school students. More recently, the LST program has been adapted for use with students at the elementary and high school levels (see LST, 2006). The program is designed to be delivered in school classroom settings.

CONTENT

Information is provided to students on drug resistance, personal self-management, and general social skills. Students are also provided with the opportunities to develop skills in each of these content areas through interactive practice (e.g., role plays). The methods of this program are designed to help students become more competent decision makers and problem solvers.

DELIVERY

The LST program has an interactive curriculum designed to be implemented by trained school personnel in classroom settings. The program is designed to be implemented across three consecutive grades (e.g., grades 6, 7, and 8). In the first academic year, students receive 15 sessions, followed by 10 and 5 sessions in the second and third years, respectively. Further booster sessions can be implemented with students in later grades.

Evaluation of a Selected (or Indicated) Prevention Program: Project Towards No Drug Abuse

The Project Towards No Drug Abuse (TND) is a program for high school students that has been tested at both the selected and indicated prevention levels (Sussman et al., 2002). Specifically, TND has been tested with students in regular high schools (at the selected level) and in alternative high schools (at the indicated level). The program is delivered to students through a series of 12 interactive classroom sessions lasting 40–50 minutes each. The sessions are designed to improve students' motivation and decision-making skills. Session content targets the prevention of drug use (e.g., use of alcohol, marijuana, or cigarettes) as well as of violent behaviors (e.g., carrying a weapon). The sessions are typically delivered by a classroom teacher who has been trained in the TND curriculum.

As described by Sussman and colleagues (2002), the early sessions of the program focus on student communication skills; misperceptions and denial associated with drug use; and negative consequences of drug use from the perspectives of the individual (i.e., adolescent), the family, and the larger social context. The middle sessions focus on providing students with both empathetic and cognitive understanding of drug abuse's negative consequences (including panel discussions of these negative consequences with ex-users or family members of users), as well as assistance in identifying healthy replacement behaviors for drug use. The last sessions focus on teaching students how to engage in appropriate social skills; presenting material on the relationship among thinking (both positive and negative), choices, and behaviors; assisting students in recognizing and avoiding violent situations; and facilitating a commitment not to use drugs. The TND program has been tested for effectiveness through a series of studies beginning in the mid-1990s.

Research Support for TND

In their initial study, Sussman, Dent, Stacy, and Craig (1998) tested the effectiveness of the TND program by assigning 21 alternative high schools to one of the following conditions (7 schools per condition): (1) nine classroom sessions; (2) nine classroom sessions plus six anti-drug activities; and (3) no prevention programming. At a 1-year follow-up, the researchers found that students in both the TND program conditions (i.e., 1 and 2) demonstrated a 25% reduction in the use of hard drugs, compared to students in the condition that did not receive the program (i.e., 3). For the students who reported using alcohol prior to receiving the program, they found reductions of 7% in use compared to students who reported using alcohol but did not receive the program. Furthermore, reductions in violent behaviors such as carrying a weapon (21%) and victimizing another person (23%) were found for male students who received TND compared to those who did not receive the program. The researchers did not find any major differences in student outcomes between the two program conditions (1 and 2) described above; thus the addition of the anti-drug activities did not enhance the effectiveness of the nine classroom sessions.

In a subsequent study, Dent, Stacy, and Craig (2001) tested the TND program with students from three regular high schools. A total of 26 classrooms among the three schools were assigned to one of two study conditions. Specifically, 13 classrooms were provided with the nine-session TND curriculum, whereas 13 classrooms were not provided with TND. At a 1-year follow-up, the researchers again found reductions in hard drug use (25%) and alcohol use (12%) for students who received the program. Reductions were also found in carrying a weapon (19%) and victimizing another person (17%) for male students who received the TND program. The results of these two studies provide support for the effectiveness of the TND program in reducing drug use and violent behaviors for students in both regular and alternative high school settings.

Core Elements of the TND Program

STRUCTURE

TND can be implemented at either the selected or indicated levels of prevention, as described above. The target groups for TND are students at alternative or regular high schools who are at risk for drug use/abuse and violent behaviors. The program is delivered to students in a classroom setting.

CONTENT

The TND classroom sessions provide students with information on, and interactive practice in, ways to prevent drug use/abuse and violent behaviors. The methods of this program are designed to improve motivation and decision-making skills for students at risk for substance abuse and violent behavior.

DELIVERY

The TND program is delivered over 12 sessions (40–50 minutes each) by teachers trained in the curriculum. The program has been implemented and tested with high school students in alternative and regular school settings.

Evaluation of an Indicated Prevention Program: Reconnecting Youth

An example of an indicated school-based prevention program designed for high school students at risk for dropping out is Reconnecting Youth (RY; Eggert et al., 2001). It is acknowledged that students at risk for school dropout typically exhibit many other risk factors, such as substance use and poor social skills. RY is composed of four major components that are designed to reconnect these students with high school as opposed to forcing them further away from it. The four components of the program include (1) having students attend a daily RY class; (2) having students engage in activities to promote school bonding; (3) increasing support and collaboration with parents; and (4) developing a school-based crisis plan. The following is a more detailed description of these four components.

The RY class is taught to a small group of high-risk students for one class period over the course of a semester (i.e., 90 days) by a teacher trained to deliver the RY curriculum. The content of the class includes teaching life skills (e.g., decision making, personal control) and ways to engage in positive peer group interaction. The school bonding component of the RY program is designed to increase the number of positive school experiences for high-risk students, as well as to promote engagement in prosocial behaviors. School bonding activities include participation in school clubs, service projects, or school-based drug-free activities. The parent involvement component of the program is designed to assist parents in reinforcing what their children are learning in the RY program, as well as to establish supportive collaboration between the RY teacher and each student's home. A positive channel of communication between school and home is important to develop, because parents with sons or daughters at risk for dropout typically receive only negative messages from school (e.g., about truancy or suspension). Finally, the crisis plan component is designed to support high-risk students who deal with issues of depression and suicidal behavior. In particular, school mental health professionals are taught how to identify suicide warning signs in students and how to support such students in receiving appropriate help. For almost two decades, the effectiveness of the RY program has been studied with high-risk students.

Research Support for RY

In an early study, Eggert, Seyl, and Nicholas (1990) assigned 124 high-risk high school students to the RY program and 140 to a control condition. At the conclusion of the study, they found that students in the RY program were more likely to stay in school, had higher grade point averages (GPAs), and demonstrated fewer problems with drug use control than students who did not receive the program. In another study (see Eggert, Thompson, Herting, Nicholas, & Dicker, 1994), the researchers assigned 101 high-risk high school students to the RY program and 158 to a control condition. They measured outcomes for all students at the conclusion of the program and during a 10-month follow-up. Students who received the RY program demonstrated increases in GPAs, self-esteem, and school bonding, as well as decreases in drug use control problems, hard drug use, and drug use progression, compared to the students who did not receive the intervention. These researchers have also found support for decreases in depression, suicide risk, stress, and anger for students who have participated in the RY program (see Eggert, Thompson, Herting, & Nicholas, 1995). Overall, the empirical findings indicate that RY is an effective indicated program for reducing substance use control problems and other negative behaviors (e.g., dropout, suicidal behavior) for high-risk high school students. In addition, there is evidence that students who receive the program experience increases in other important areas, such as academic performance (GPA), self-esteem, and school bonding.

Core Elements of the RY Program

STRUCTURE

RY is an indicated prevention program, and the target group consists of high school students at risk for school dropout. The central program component is delivered to students in a classroom setting. Other program components include student school bonding activities, strengthening parent collaboration, and training school personnel in crisis management.

CONTENT

The RY class provides students with life skills information and practice, as well as positive peer group interaction. The methods of this program are designed to improve decision making, self-control, self-esteem, and interpersonal communication skills for at-risk students.

DELIVERY

The content of the RY class is delivered by specially trained teachers using an interactive curriculum. The program has been implemented and tested with high-risk high school students.

Evaluation of a Tiered Program: Adolescent Transitions Program

Up to this point, we have focused on programs that were generally designed to target one level of prevention. The Adolescent Transitions Program (ATP), however, is a prevention program designed to address student and family needs at multiple levels (Dishion & Kavanagh, 2003). That is, the program is tiered so that interventions occur at universal, selected, and indicated levels, as required. This prevention program is slightly different from some of the others reviewed, because there is a strong focus on providing family-based services that are linked to the school setting.

The *universal* prevention component is termed the Family Resource Room (FRR). The FRR is a specially designated room in a school that is staffed by a full-time mental health professional (e.g., a family counselor or social worker) and is stocked with a range of parenting and family resources (e.g., videos, books, brochures). The major goals of the FRR are to connect parents positively with their children's school environment, as well as to provide various means of support for positive parenting practices. Many different types of information and interactive resources are offered to parents by the FRR staff; these include assisting parents in promoting positive behavior (e.g., academic, social) in their children, as well as a structured 6-week parent–child education curriculum designed to promote both child and parent success.

If warranted, the FRR staff can refer a family to the *selected* prevention component: the Family Check-Up (FCU), which is a three-step process of family assessment conducted by a mental health professional. The specific goals of the FCU are to assist in determining positive areas of family life that should be maintained, as well as challenging areas that are appropriate for intervention. The specific steps of the FCU include providing an initial interview to explain the FCU process to the family, conducting a comprehensive assessment of family members, and providing a family feedback session to explain assessment results and referral suggestions.

If the members of a family require intervention beyond the FCU, they are provided with a Menu of Services, which is an *indicated* level of prevention. Its goal is to provide families with a range of professional services from which they can choose the ones that best meet their needs. The types of professional services offered include family therapy, parenting groups, and case management services. The ATP as a whole has been studied for its effectiveness with adolescents and families, and we describe this research next.

Research Support for ATP

Dishion and Kavanagh (2003) state that the ATP is based on the empirical findings of many research studies indicating that family-based interventions serve to decrease problem behaviors in adolescents. The findings of overall effectiveness for the ATP have been emerging during the past few years. For example, Dishion, Kavanagh, Schneigher, Nelson, and Kaufman (2002) followed 672 students from the 6th to 9th grades attending three public middle schools. All of these students received the FRR (universal) component of the ATP, whereas mainly high-risk students received the selected and indicated components of the ATP. The researchers' findings indicated that in 9th grade, both typically developing and high-risk students who received the intervention showed reductions in substance use. They suggested that these findings point to the effectiveness of the FRR universal component, as the typically developing students only received this part of the ATP.

In a more recent study, Stormshak, Dishion, Light, and Yasui (2005) followed 584 students in four public middle schools over a period of 3 years. Each school integrated an FRR, and also provided selected and indicated interventions consistent with the ATP model. They found that students and their families who had more contact with the FRR over the middle school years showed reductions in problem behaviors (e.g., poor classroom behavior, tobacco use, poor academic achievement) as perceived by their teachers. In sum, the findings from these studies are encouraging regarding the effectiveness of the ATP for preventing and reducing substance use and problem behavior in middle school students. We anticipate that more research supporting the effectiveness of the ATP will be forthcoming in the near future.

Core Elements of the ATP

STRUCTURE

ATP is a multilevel prevention program, and the target groups are middle school students and their families. The program is designed to be delivered in schools and/or community clinics, depending on whether the intervention takes place at the universal, selected, or indicated level.

CONTENT

At the universal prevention level, information is provided to parents and their children on such topics as positive parenting practices and assessing student competencies (e.g., social, academic). For the selected prevention level, families are provided with the FCU, which assists family members in determining which areas of family life are working well and which need improvement. Finally, at the indicated prevention level, parents are provided with a Menu of Services from which to choose, in order to receive professional assistance for family problem areas.

DELIVERY

Services at the universal level of the ATP are delivered in the school's FRR by a mental health professional, whereas services at the selected and indicated levels are delivered in school or community clinic settings by mental health professionals. The program has been tested for use with middle school students and their families. At each level of intervention, this program provides a range of family-based approaches.

Summary of Research-Based Prevention Programs

As the review above has made clear, there are effective substance abuse programs for each prevention level depicted in Figure 4.1. Programs such as LST are designed to target all students (i.e., they are universal prevention programs). Programs such as TND and RY, however, are designed to target specific groups of students at the selected and indicated prevention levels, respectively. Tiered programs such as the ATP are designed to provide interventions to students at each prevention level.

Beyond the four programs described here, there are several other substance abuse prevention programs that have been endorsed by national government agencies such as the NIDA and the Center for Substance Abuse Prevention (CSAP). Therefore, we recommend that school mental health professionals critically review and compare the available substance abuse prevention programs prior to choosing one for their school. In addition to selecting a program, school professionals will need to make informed planning decisions prior to implementing the program in their school setting.

EVALUATING THE DRUG ABUSE RESISTANCE EDUCATION PROGRAM

We assume that most school mental health professionals are familiar with the Drug Abuse Resistance Education (D.A.R.E.) program, because it is the most widely implemented drug abuse prevention program in schools throughout the United States (Clayton, Cattarello, & Johnstone, 1996; Ennett, Tobler, Ringwalt, & Flewelling, 1994). In fact, it is estimated that between 50% and 80% of school districts across the nation implement some version of this program (Ennett et al., 1994; Komro et al., 2004). We have chosen not to discuss this program in the section above, because although it is highly popular and widely used, the available research findings suggest that it is not very effective (Clayton, Leukefeld, Harrington, & Cattarello, 1996). Therefore, we have chosen to discuss and evaluate this program separately from the research-based prevention programs.

In contrast to the programs described above, which were developed and tested within the context of research studies, the D.A.R.E. program was originally developed through a joint collaboration of the Los Angeles Unified School District and the Los Angeles Police Department. In 1983, these two agencies launched D.A.R.E. in order to teach students in their last year of elementary school how to resist engaging in drug use and violent behavior (Koch, 1994). The program has also been adapted for use with secondary students (see Koch, 1994), but our discussion here focuses on the elementary school version, because the vast majority of rigorous evaluation studies have been conducted with students who received this version (Clayton, Cattarello, et al., 1996; Ennett et al., 1994). In addition, the original D.A.R.E. curriculum has been updated since its introduction; one such update is called the D.A.R.E. Plus program. However, we found only one evaluation study of the D.A.R.E. Plus program—by Komro and colleagues (2004)—and it focused on violence rather than substance abuse. In sum, our discussion of D.A.R.E. in this section is based on the original version of the program delivered to students in the last year of elementary school.

D.A.R.E. is a universal substance abuse prevention program that involves a 17-session curriculum implemented by a uniformed police officer in the classroom setting (Koch, 1994); each session lasts approximately 1 hour. Topics covered include drug use and consequences, resisting drug use, managing stress, media influences, and resisting pressure to join a gang. Students learn the material by being provided educational information as well as engaging in interactive exercises (e.g., role plays). Police officers are taught to deliver the curriculum to students by attending 80 hours of a D.A.R.E.-specific training course (Clayton, Leukefeld, et al., 1996).

Evaluation Studies of D.A.R.E.

In one of the most comprehensive evaluations of D.A.R.E. to date, Ennett and her colleagues (1994) identified eight studies in which D.A.R.E. had been implemented as a universal prevention program with elementary school students. They then compared these D.A.R.E. studies to research on the outcomes of other drug abuse prevention programs that targeted students of a similar age. For comparison purposes, they grouped programs into one of three categories: D.A.R.E., noninteractive, or interactive. As described by Tobler (1992), *noninteractive* programs focus on providing students with information or knowledge that is delivered by an adult expert, with few (if any) learning exercises. In contrast, *interactive* programs focus on improving students' social competencies (e.g., social skills, decision making, problem solving) through the use of learning exercises such as role plays, in which both adults and peers can deliver. In general, interactive substance abuse prevention programs tend to have better outcomes than noninteractive programs do (Tobler, 1992).

The outcomes for D.A.R.E., noninteractive, and interactive programs were compared across studies, immediately after students had been exposed to one of these programs, in the following areas: knowledge of drugs, attitudes toward drug use, social skills, self-esteem, and drug use (Ennett et al., 1994). The researchers found that of the three program types, interactive programs demonstrated the best outcomes in all four areas. The D.A.R.E. program had its best outcome on students' knowledge of drugs, but this knowledge level was still lower than in the interactive programs. D.A.R.E. outcomes for students' attitudes toward drug use and social skills were only slightly better than those for noninteractive programs and were much lower than those for interactive programs.

Finally, across all three program types, D.A.R.E. demonstrated the poorest outcomes for students' actual drug use immediately following completion of the program.

Clayton and his colleagues (Clayton, Cattarello, et al., 1996; Lynam et al., 1999) have conducted two long-term evaluation studies of D.A.R.E. by tracking students who either received or did not receive the program in grade 6. In their first study, Clayton, Cattarello, and colleagues (1996) assessed students in 23 schools who received D.A.R.E. and students in 8 other schools who "received a drug education unit as part of the health curriculum" (p. 307). All of the students in this study were assessed before the D.A.R.E. program or the drug education unit began in grade 6, after completion of the program or unit, and once a year thereafter for the next 4 years. Students were assessed in areas that the D.A.R.E. program attempts to target, including drug use; attitudes toward specific drugs (i.e., alcohol, cigarettes, and marijuana); general attitudes toward drugs; ability to resist negative pressure from peers; and perceived use of alcohol, cigarettes, and marijuana by peers.

In grade 7, students who received D.A.R.E. demonstrated better outcomes than the students who did not receive the program in the following areas: attitudes toward drugs (general and specific); ability to resist negative peer pressure; and perceived drug use of peers (Clayton, Cattarello, et al., 1996). However, no differences were found between the two groups at this point for use of alcohol, cigarettes, or marijuana. In addition, the differences found in grade 7 for the D.A.R.E. students did not last over time, as both groups were similar on all measures at grade 10. Of particular significance was that no differences in reported drug use were found between the two groups of students in grade 10, even though drug use/abuse resistance is one of the main goals of D.A.R.E.

In a subsequent study, Lynam and colleagues (1999) tracked and assessed the same two groups of students described above, 10 years after the D.A.R.E. program was delivered in elementary school. These students were now young adults between the ages of 19 and 21. They were assessed on use of specific drugs (i.e., alcohol, cigarettes, marijuana, illicit drugs); positive and negative expectancies of drug use; and the ability to resist negative pressure from peers. The researchers found no differences between the two groups on any of these outcome measures. In particular, the level of past drug use reported at age 20 was not related to whether these young adults received D.A.R.E. in grade 6 or not. Other researchers who have conducted long-term evaluation studies of D.A.R.E. have found similar results (see Dukes, Stein, & Ullman, 1997; Dukes, Ullman, & Stein, 1996).

Core Elements of D.A.R.E.

Structure

D.A.R.E. is a universal prevention program. As described above, the target audience for the original version of D.A.R.E. is students in the last year of elementary school; the program has also been adapted for use with secondary students. An updated version (D.A.R.E. Plus) has been developed but awaits thorough evaluation. It is designed to be delivered in a classroom setting.

Content

The topics covered include drug use and consequences, resisting drug use, managing stress, media influences, and resisting pressure to join a gang. Students are given educational information, as well as opportunities to engage in role plays and other interactive exercises.

Delivery

The program curriculum (which consists of 17 sessions lasting about 1 hour each) is delivered to students by a specially trained uniformed police officer in a classroom setting. The vast majority of outcome studies have been conducted on the elementary school version. Research is needed on the D.A.R.E. program for secondary students, as well as the updated D.A.R.E. Plus curriculum.

Why Is D.A.R.E. So Popular?

At this point our readers may be asking, "Why is D.A.R.E. so popular, even though research findings don't support its effectiveness?" This is an excellent question. Clayton, Leukefeld, and colleagues (1996) suggest that D.A.R.E. has been popular in schools for a number of reasons, one of which has been continuous federal funding. Specifically, D.A.R.E. was singled out for federal support in the 1986 Drug-Free Schools and Communities Act, and this support has continued through the more recent Safe and Drug-Free Schools and Communities Act (Clayton, Leukefeld, et al., 1996). Another reason for D.A.R.E.'s widespread use is that several factors have made it attractive to influential stakeholders at the community level, including police officers, teachers, administrators, and parents. First, the fact that a uniformed police officer is placed in a school as part of the D.A.R.E. program serves to promote positive community relations between local schools and police departments. Second, teachers are not required to teach the D.A.R.E. curriculum because it is delivered by a police officer, and this frees them for other teaching responsibilities. Third, administrators are influenced by the reactions of teachers and parents, and all three of these groups tend to have positive reactions to the D.A.R.E. program. Donnermeyer and Wurschmidt (1997) found that a sample of 286 elementary school teachers and principals positively rated the quality of the D.A.R.E. program and its impact on students. Finally, teachers, administrators, and parents all perceive schools to be safer when D.A.R.E. police officers are present (Clayton, Leukefeld, et al., 1996).

In short, the D.A.R.E. program receives a lot of support from its key stakeholders in local communities, as well as continuous funding from the federal government. These combined factors have served to overshadow the lack of research evidence for the effectiveness of this program. Other substance abuse prevention programs that have research support for their effectiveness do not receive the same amount of positive governmental or social support as D.A.R.E. We believe that these are the major reasons why D.A.R.E.

continues to be implemented in large numbers of schools across the United States, even though more effective substance abuse prevention programs exist.

PLANNING FOR IMPLEMENTATION OF A SUBSTANCE ABUSE PREVENTION PROGRAM

We have found from practical experience that at the end of a typical school year, school personnel are bombarded with numerous proposals for programs to implement in their schools the following fall. These programs range from reading curricula to substance abuse prevention programs. We have also found that school personnel often choose programs on the basis of such factors as the attractiveness of the packaging and materials, not the actual demonstrated effectiveness of the programs. Other questions commonly overlooked by school personnel in deciding to implement a program are "Is our school ready to implement this program?" and "What are the steps needed to implement a prevention program successfully?"

Robertson and colleagues (2003) suggest that communities consider four planning guidelines prior to implementing a substance abuse prevention program. We have revised these guidelines for the school setting as follows:

1. *School personnel need to know the actual severity of the problem (actual student substance use and abuse, related problem behaviors, and associated risk factors).* We have found that school administration tend to rely on casual observations of students or anecdotal information to determine the severity of problem behaviors in their school, as opposed to using existing data (e.g., number of referrals for substance problems in a school year) or collecting data (e.g., conducting a needs assessment).

2. *School personnel need to determine whether the school is ready to implement a substance abuse prevention program.* We have seen many examples of motivated school personnel who implement a program at the beginning of the school year, only to have it fizzle toward the end of the year due to decreased staff enthusiasm, active staff resistance, or other factors.

3. *School personnel need to review the existing programs in their school or surrounding community, and to target specific areas of need that are not being addressed by those programs.* For example, it does not make much sense to implement a universal substance abuse prevention program if a school already has a similar program in place and it is working.

4. *School personnel should make connections with relevant community organizations that can provide resources and support for the long-term implementation of the program.* Imagine that you want to staff an FRR similar to the one in the ATP as described above, but your school does not have funding for the necessary personnel. One possible solution is to develop a collaborative relationship with a local college or university with graduate programs in psychology or social work. Such programs are often searching for practicum sites for their students. Your school's FRR could be developed as a training site and

staffed by a graduate student, which would solve your personnel problem and at the same time provide valuable training for the student.

Now let's take a closer look at each of these major planning guidelines.

What Is the Severity of the Problem?

In order to answer the question posed by the first guideline, school mental health professionals need to assess and understand the actual severity of student substance use in their school. They should also assess the severity of related problem behaviors (e.g., disruptive behavior, truancies) and associated risk factors (e.g., the availability of various drugs in the local community). School mental health professionals can use two major methods to assess these factors; one is to examine preexisting data, and the other is to collect local school and community data. In fact, the most comprehensive method is to use both existing data and original data to assess the problem's severity. Of course, assessment procedures are limited by the resources available to the school and its personnel. Therefore, as you read this section, think about the most realistic way to conduct a severity assessment in your school setting.

Using Existing Data

As we have noted throughout this book, many sources of data on adolescent substance use are available at the local and national levels, generally free of charge. For example, we have described the national data collected in the Monitoring the Future (MTF) studies and the NSDUH in Chapter 1. To recap briefly, the MTF research annually provides national data on the drug use patterns of students in grades 8, 10, and 12; the NSDUH provides drug use estimates for the civilian population of children through adults in the nation, as well as individual state estimates on drug use. The CSAP hosts a useful website for locating additional sources of national data on adolescent substance use (see "Chapter Resources"). Such data can be useful to school mental health professionals for purposes of comparison to the student body in their school.

There may also be valuable sources of data on adolescent substance use rates in a particular state. In addition to the NSDUH state-level data (see above), many state offices of substance abuse or mental health across the country track the prevalence of adolescence substance use at state and county levels. For example, in the past few years the state in which both of us authors reside (Utah) began conducting a statewide survey of substance use rates, other related health behaviors, and risk and protective factors for students across the K–12 spectrum. This survey provides valuable information at the state, county, and school district levels on substance use rates and risk–protective factors for students at different grades; it also compares the state's use rates to national norms. We suggest checking with other states' offices of substance abuse or mental health to determine whether such data exist for those states.

Schools also routinely collect their own data on student problem behavior. School records such as office discipline referrals, suspensions, and referrals to community agencies (e.g., substance abuse treatment centers) can be examined as sources of direct or indirect information on student substance use severity. For example, school mental health professionals could easily tally the number of students who were counseled for substance-abuse-related issues (while maintaining student confidentiality) over the past 1–3 school years. These types of data would provide information on the severity of student substance use in the school, as well as information indicating whether the problem is getting worse (i.e., an increase in students seen for substance abuse counseling). In addition, Web-based data organization systems such as the School-Wide Information System (SWIS) have been designed to track problem behaviors, including alcohol and drug abuse, across school academic years. More information on SWIS can be found at its website (*www.swis.org*). In sum, we suggest that school mental health professionals think about which types of data are already available to them and how these data can be used to assist in determining the severity of student substance use.

Collecting Original Data

A more challenging prospect is collecting original data on a school's student body. Some schools have developed their own surveys to assess the health-related behaviors of their students, whereas other schools have administered standardized surveys to their students. Some of the potential obstacles to collecting original data include time, expense, and expertise. That is, collecting data takes personnel time; it typically costs money; and someone with expertise in survey development is needed to assist in the process. If school mental health professionals decide to develop and administer their own survey, we strongly suggest consulting with someone in the local community (e.g., a university professor, state office personnel) who has expertise in survey development, administration, and interpretation. All too often, time and money are wasted on surveys that were poorly developed and thus do not provide the information desired, or the data cannot be summarized in a manner that allows school professionals to answer questions of greatest concern (e.g., "What is the substance most frequently used by our students?").

Another option for original data collection is to administer a standardized survey to students. One example is the Communities That Care Youth Survey (Arthur, Hawkins, Pollard, Catalano, & Baglioni, 2002), which has 121 items and measures 29 risk and protective factor domains and health-related behaviors (e.g., substance use, violent acts). The survey is designed to be administered to students ranging in age from 11 to 18 in a 50-minute classroom period. It has been tested with a large sample of students in grades 6, 8, and 11, and is considered an effective instrument for assessing secondary students' health-related behaviors (see Arthur et al., 2002). The survey and supporting materials are available free of charge from the National Clearinghouse for Alcohol and Drug Information (NCADI; see "Chapter Resources"). Using standardized instruments such as this one can save school time and expense. In addition, we again recommend visiting the

CSAP website, which provides further information on assessment instruments. After collecting and interpreting data on the severity of student substance use in a school, the next step is to determine whether the school is ready to implement a prevention program.

Is the School Ready to Implement a Substance Abuse Prevention Program?

Determining whether a school is ready to implement a substance abuse prevention program is a step that is typically overlooked. Examining school readiness is important, however, because school personnel can implement an effective program poorly when the larger system (i.e., school, staff, and parents) is not ready. Edwards, Jumper-Thurman, Plested, Oetting, and Swanson (2000) developed a nine-stage *community readiness model* (CRM), which indicates both how aware communities are of a specific problem and how ready they are to implement a program for dealing with the problem. Edwards and her colleagues discuss the model in terms of communities; however, we believe that this model is easily adapted to schools, as they are small communities unto themselves. In our description of the CRM below, we have therefore revised each stage for relevancy in a school context. As you read through each stage, try to determine how ready your school is to implement a substance abuse prevention program.

1. *No awareness*. The school and its personnel do not recognize that a substance use/abuse problem exists in the student body when such a problem does exist. School personnel in this stage may state "Our students don't have problems with drugs."

2. *Denial*. The majority of personnel in a school do not think that a student substance use/abuse problem exists; however, a minority of personnel do recognize the potential for such a problem. For example, the counselors are seeing increasing numbers of students for substance-abuse-related problems, but the larger faculty does not view substance abuse as an issue that needs to be addressed. School personnel in this stage may state, "Only a few students in the school have problems with substances; it's not a big deal."

3. *Vague awareness*. There is general agreement among school personnel that a student substance use/abuse problem exists, but little motivation for actually dealing with the problem. School personnel in this stage may state, "Students in our school have problems with drugs, but we can't do anything about it," or "We don't have the time or money to deal with student substance abuse in our school."

4. *Preplanning*. Some school personnel clearly recognize that a student substance use/abuse problem exists and needs to be addressed. A committee of concerned school personnel may have been formed to discuss the problem, but concrete steps to address the problem have not yet been identified. A committee member in this stage may state, "Student substance abuse is a problem, and we need to deal with it."

5. *Preparation*. A committee of school personnel discusses the practicalities involved in addressing a student substance use/abuse problem in the school. Members of the committee are motivated to address the problem; assignments are made; and

resources are assessed. Other personnel in the school are in general support of the committee's efforts to address the problem.

6. *Initiation.* Initial action has been taken by a committee to address the problem. This may include having in-service training sessions or something similar. Members of the committee express high levels of enthusiasm for moving the initiative forward; the larger school community is generally supportive of the initiative taken by the committee; and others may become involved.

7. *Stabilization.* A substance abuse prevention program has been implemented in the school and is viewed as being stable within the school community. School personnel, including administration, are generally supportive of the program as implemented. Any program modifications, based on program evaluation, are not being considered in this stage.

8. *Confirmation and expansion.* The original substance abuse prevention program has become integrated into the school setting; staff and students can easily utilize its services. The program has also been evaluated, and the data are being used to make decisions about program modifications and expansion. In addition, interventions at the selected or indicated levels of prevention may be initiated, based on data from the original program. The school community continues to provide general support for the program.

9. *Professionalization.* The substance abuse prevention program is targeting the problem at multiple levels of prevention: universal, selected, and indicated. School personnel are much better informed about the problem (e.g., prevalence, risk factors) than at earlier stages. The program is being run efficiently by trained school staff members, and data from program evaluation are used to make modifications as necessary. The school community continues to provide general support for the program.

The nine-stage CRM provides guidelines not only for assessing a school community's readiness to implement a substance abuse prevention program, but also for considering what actions need to be taken to move through each stage. Edwards and her colleagues (2000) recommend that these actions be based on ideas both from the committee and from the larger community in which the program was implemented. For example, the committee formed to address the student substance use/abuse problem can work with personnel in the larger school community to develop strategies that will increase school readiness. The goal is to create strategies which are realistic and appropriate for a particular school setting. Let's say that a committee determines its school to be in the *denial* stage. Working with the larger school faculty, the committee can then plan activities (e.g., presenting relevant information at an in-service training session) to increase school personnel's awareness that a student substance use/abuse problem exists. Strategies for the *preplanning* stage may include providing specific assignments to committee members (e.g., gathering student substance abuse data) that will move them from abstract to concrete program planning. The main point here is that school personnel should develop readiness strategies at each stage that will facilitate movement to the next stage. We have provided a chart (Figure 4.2) that our readers can use to assess a school's

Stage of readiness	Reasons why your school *is* or *is not* in this stage	Strategies for your school to move through this stage
No awareness		
Denial		
Vague awareness		
Preplanning		
Preparation		
Initiation		
Stabilization		
Confirmation and expansion		
Professionalism		

FIGURE 4.2. School Readiness Form.

Based on the community readiness model (CRM) in Edwards, Jumper-Thurman, Plested, Oetting, and Swanson (2000). From Jason J. Burrow-Sanchez and Leanne S. Hawken (2007). Copyright by The Guilford Press. Permission to photocopy this figure is granted to purchasers of this book for personal use only (see copyright page for details).

readiness to implement a prevention program, as well as to identify strategies for moving through each stage.

What Are the Existing Gaps in Services for Students?

Another important planning guideline is to review the programs currently being offered by a school for preventing substance abuse or mental health issues. The goal of this step is not only to identify existing services, but, more importantly, to identify gaps in existing services for students. This will ensure that programs are not duplicated and that all students in the prevention triangle receive services. For example, a school may have implemented an effective prevention program for substance abuse at the universal level, but services may be nonexistent for students at the selected or indicated levels. Following this planning guideline will provide a good idea of which services are most needed in a school.

In What Ways Can the School Collaborate with the Local Community?

A final step is to determine in what ways the school can collaborate with the local community in implementing a substance abuse prevention program. Collaboration with the community provides not only initial external support for the program, but additional resources that may be needed to ensure the program's long-term success. For example, if it appears that community referrals to substance abuse treatment centers will be needed as part of the program, establishing relationships with two or three local treatment agencies will be beneficial. As mentioned above, local colleges and universities may also be able to provide personnel, in the form of students, who can assist in implementing the program. We encourage school mental health professionals to brainstorm all the community agencies or programs that could potentially serve as resources for the implementation and sustainability of a school-based prevention program. Once a substantial list of agencies or programs has been compiled, three or four of these should be contacted. If the first few contacts do not work out, others should be made. We are certain that some of these community resources will be willing to collaborate on the implementation of a substance abuse prevention program.

CASE EXAMPLE

Jalen Singh was a school psychologist at Hunter Middle School, which is located in an urban area with a population of just over 1,000 students. Jalen was increasingly concerned about an apparent increase in the use of inhalants by Hunter's students. This increase seemed to have coincided with a local news story that highlighted the problem of inhalant use in the area, but also provided the audience examples of different ways teens were getting high. Several students had been referred to the office for acting out following lunch or break times, and several of the referrals mentioned suspected drug use (e.g., "The student was out of it . . . seemed like he was on something"). In addition, the school custodian had recently found several spray paint canisters and glue containers behind one of the dumpsters.

Jalen mentioned his concern to other school personnel, and many echoed his concern but didn't know how to address the problem. They mentioned that they would like all students to receive some type of information about the negative effects of inhalants and other drugs, but that certain students, as indicated by office discipline referrals and other data, could use more intensive interventions related to substance abuse. Some members of the school staff, however, were not very concerned and felt that the problem had been "blown out of proportion" by the local media.

The first step Jalen took was to gather additional information on the extent of the problem. He gathered all of the office discipline referrals for drug-related offenses; he also summarized the data on the number of students he had individually seen for substance-use-related behaviors. Since Jalen had worked at Hunter Middle School for over 8 years, he was able to gather sufficient information to show that there had been clear increases in both data categories. He also noted that referrals to outside agencies for substance abuse treatment, although still low, had increased over the past 5 years.

With these data in hand, Jalen spoke with both the school principal and his supervisor at the district level, to gain their support for collecting additional data to document the extent of the problem. He felt that if he could gather more support for his concern, he would be able to convince the faculty that a universal substance abuse prevention program should be implemented. After this meeting with his administrators, Jalen was given permission to administer the Communities That Care Youth Survey (Arthur et al., 2002). He spoke with the teachers and determined that the best time to administer the survey was during the advisory period; because this was only a 30-minute period, it would need to be administered across two sessions.

Following administration of the Communities That Care Youth Survey, Jalen summarized the data and determined that over 40% of the student population had used inhalants or some other type of drug in the past 6 months. These data alone were enough to cause alarm among the staff. At the next staff meeting, Jalen shared the data and asked the faculty to vote on whether or not a universal prevention program was needed to address drug abuse at Hunter Middle School. Based on the research he had read about systems change, he figured that if he could get at least an 80% "buy-in" from the staff, it meant that enough staff members would be interested in implementing a universal intervention. Jalen asked staff members to vote anonymously as to whether or not they would help implement such an intervention. Much to his surprise, over 88% of the staff agreed both that a universal intervention was needed and that they would be willing to help with it. In the faculty meeting, Jalen also mentioned that he would be working more intensively, using selected interventions, with students who were at higher risk or who had already been referred to the office for drug-related offenses.

Following the faculty votes, Jalen worked with the student study team to determine which universal prevention program would be most appropriate for their school. A counselor in a neighboring middle school mentioned that her school had implemented LST as a universal intervention and had seen significant reductions in drug use over a 4-year period. As Jalen reviewed the LST curriculum, he liked the fact that it was research-based and had been tested in middle school settings.

After reviewing the LST curriculum, Jalen determined that it would be a good universal prevention program, but that he would really like to involve parents more in preventing substance abuse. Several teachers had expressed concerns that a universal prevention program would not be truly effective unless parents were hearing the same messages and giving these to their kids. Jalen searched the Internet for more information on substance abuse prevention programs, and found descriptions of and research on the ATP. He liked the idea of the FRR mentioned in these descriptions, but was unsure how he would get the resources to implement one in his school. He was mainly concerned that with his current duties, he would be unable himself to devote the necessary time and attention to running an FRR.

During his next meeting with all of the counselors and school psychologists in the district, Jalen mentioned the goal of developing an FRR and his concern about being able to staff it on a regular basis. He mentioned that he had talked to his principal and that she had agreed to provide him with a room adjacent to the library, but that he still needed help with resources to staff the room, as there was no room in the budget for additional personnel. Many of the school psychologists at his meeting mentioned that they had been asked by a local university to supervise students in school psychology practica. Several of the counselors in the meeting had also been approached to provide supervision, but there were more students who needed placements than either the psychologists or the counselors could supervise. After this meeting, Jalen contacted faculty members at the local university and determined that they were indeed looking for school counseling and school psychology practicum sites and were interested in providing their students with experience in school-based prevention programming. The university committed itself to providing at least two students per year who each would be required to work 15 hours in the school.

With all of these resources in place, Jalen helped design and staff the FRR and trained teachers how to implement the LST program. He also worked with 10 students across the school year who needed selected interventions. These students were given additional academic support (i.e., after-school tutoring); they also met weekly with Jalen to learn more intensive problem-solving skills, as well as to practice demonstrating these skills. Within 1 year of implementing the universal and selected interventions, Hunter Middle School experienced a 40% reduction in office discipline referrals—not only for substance-abuse-related offenses, but also for other student offenses (e.g., defiance, extreme disruption). Based on these initial results, the school staff and administration provided strong support for continuing the universal and selected prevention programs during the following school year.

CHAPTER SUMMARY

The goals of prevention programs are to keep a potential problem from occurring or to keep an existing problem from getting worse. School-based programs are designed to target one or more levels of prevention: universal, selected, and indicated. NIDA has developed a set of prevention principles based on decades of research in this area. School mental health professionals should examine how well any existing substance abuse prevention programs and any future programs they plan to implement meet the NIDA guidelines. Many research-based prevention programs are available for school professionals to choose from; the structure, content, and delivery of some of these programs have been reviewed in this chapter, to provide a model for how school professionals can evaluate programs they are considering. Factors that should be considered by school professionals before implementing a prevention program include the severity of the problem at their school, existing gaps in services for students, and the readiness of their school to implement such a program. Finally, a case example has illustrated the steps taken by a school psychologist to implement substance abuse prevention programming in his school.

CHAPTER RESOURCES

Center for Substance Abuse Prevention (CSAP)

prevention.samhsa.gov

As noted in the chapter text, this website provides lots of great resources on the topic of prevention, as well as a searchable database for locating research-based substance abuse prevention programs.

SAMHSA Model Programs

modelprograms.samhsa.gov

This website provides a listing of evidence-based programs that SAMHSA terms "model programs," based on the criteria listed on the site. The listing includes a range of prevention and reduction programs targeting substance abuse and mental health problems.

National Institute on Drug Abuse (NIDA)

www.nida.nih.gov

This website is a great resource for all types of information related to drug abuse. It contains specific links for students, parents, and school professionals. The publication *Preventing Drug Abuse among Children and Adolescents: A Research-Based Guide for Parents, Educators, and Community Leaders* can be downloaded from this site.

National Clearinghouse for Alcohol and Drug Information (NCADI)

ncadi.samhsa.gov

This government-hosted website provides thousands of resources on topics related to substance abuse and mental health, which can be directly ordered from the site. Most of these materials can be obtained free of charge.

American Academy of Pediatrics

www.aap.org/family/subabuse.htm

This site provides information for parents about what they need to know and can do about preventing substance abuse in their children.

American Council for Drug Education

www.acde.org

This website, hosted by Phoenix House, provides a lot of information and materials for teens, parents, and educators on the topic of substance abuse.

Parents: The Anti-Drug

www.theantidrug.com

This website is sponsored by the National Youth Anti-Drug Media Campaign and provides information on substance abuse topics for parents, as well as students and school professionals.

5

Individual Interventions

Erin M. Ingoldsby *and* David Ehrman

The goal of this chapter is to review individual intervention approaches for substance-using students. We review the essential components for working directly or indirectly with such students—from those who are "experimenting" to those who are demonstrating significant drug abuse. First, let's describe what we mean by *individual interventions*. These are interventions that involve direct counseling (one-on-one work with a student), with the goal of helping the student to reduce or cease substance use. As a school mental health professional, you may be the person who initially learns about the student's drug use and identifies the need for intervention, or you may be informed about it during or after the student's participation in a treatment program. You might take on a number of roles in an intervention, including meeting with a student to talk about substance use patterns and assessing whether the student is ready to make a change; helping the student, family, and other school professionals identify intervention resources; supporting interventions occurring in outpatient or inpatient settings; or conducting counseling directly with the student. It is important, then, to be aware of the ways that adolescent substance use is effectively treated, in order to know what you and your school can do and how you can help.

Whether a school mental health professional should plan to do an intervention program with a substance-using student depends on a number of factors, including the

Erin M. Ingoldsby, PhD, is Assistant Professor in the Department of Psychology at the University of Utah. **David Ehrman, BA,** University of Utah.

school's policy on substance use problems and the severity of the problem. When the student's substance use is more serious, ideal treatment involves many different contributors to the intervention process—the adolescent, family members, therapist or treatment program providers, school counselors, teachers, and others—all working together with coordinated goals. Such "continuity of care" has been associated with the best long-term outcomes (Williams & Chang, 2000). However, this type of comprehensive program isn't always feasible for school personnel, and students most often receive treatment for drug problems outside the school setting. We spend some time describing the types of individually based interventions that are commonly used in different settings, including inpatient/hospital-based and residential programs, outpatient programs, and family treatment. The objective is to help school mental health professionals understand what students go through as they receive treatment, and how these professionals can support treatment efforts, even when they are not providing direct intervention. For example, we offer some thoughts about working with treatment agencies to help a student make the transition from a residential treatment program back into the school setting.

In a situation in which a student's drug use is just beginning to become a noticeable problem, several early intervention strategies may be used by a school mental health professional. At present, well-tested interventions that are specifically designed for school personnel to treat student substance use problems are rare. Therefore, we draw on programs and materials from promising new treatments being tested in outpatient clinics. As we go along, we note critical components in intervening with a substance-using adolescent, including the importance of building connection, trust, and motivation with the adolescent; working successfully with families and other involved professionals; making informed referral and treatment decisions for students with co-occurring conditions, such as attention-deficit/hyperactivity disorder (ADHD) or depression; and supporting the educational and learning needs of these adolescents. A case example is used to help illustrate important concepts and intervention strategies. The chapter ends with a list of resources for school personnel interested in learning more about individual interventions.

TYPES OF INDIVIDUAL INTERVENTIONS FOR SUBSTANCE-USING ADOLESCENTS

Compared to the treatments available for substance-using adults and the research on these treatments, up until the last few decades there were very few treatments specifically developed for adolescents, and even fewer studies testing how well these treatments work (Deas & Thomas, 2001). More recently, some studies have tried to address the unique treatment needs of substance-using adolescents (Muck et al., 2001). Thanks to this research, and to recommendations from adolescent substance use experts in multiple areas (e.g., psychiatry, psychology, juvenile justice), much more information about effective treatment strategies is now available. Elsewhere, interested school mental health professionals can find reports that describe the best treatment models and strategies (American Academy of Child and Adolescent Psychiatry [AACAP], 2005; Center for Substance Abuse Treatment [CSAT], 1999a, 1999b, 1999c).

How Are Substance-Using Adolescents Currently Treated?

The reality is that most students who try drugs, or even use drugs recreationally, do not receive any treatment. One reason for this is that many students either use drugs only occasionally or, even if they use more regularly, naturally tend to decrease their level of use as they grow into early adulthood (Brown, 2001). Yet even among adolescents with very serious drug use and disorders, relatively few end up in treatment programs. Of the 1.4 million students between the ages of 12 and 17 estimated to have problems with illicit drugs, only about 10% receive any treatment (Dennis & McGeary, 1999). For treated adolescents, outpatient programs were the most common type of treatment (69%), followed by intensive outpatient (11%), long-term residential (9%), short-term residential (6%), and other treatment programs (6%, including inpatient hospitalization and detox programs) (Muck et al., 2001).

The way substance abuse is treated depends a great deal on the treatment orientation of the service provider. *Treatment orientation* includes core beliefs about the factors and processes contributing to drug use and addiction, as well as about the best ways to treat these problems. Although the treatment orientations of adolescent programs may vary, most share some components. The long-term goal for most interventions is *abstinence* (i.e., no drug use). In many programs, abstinence is a requirement for being in treatment. However, from a practical standpoint, *harm reduction* (i.e., decreasing the potential harm associated with risky behaviors such as drug use, without attempting to prohibit the behaviors) may be the implicit short-term goal in treatment (AACAP, 2005). From this perspective, a positive outcome of treatment might mean that the student (1) has reduced his or her drug use; (2) has reduced risky behavior that was associated with drug use; (3) doesn't relapse as often; or (4) has improved in other areas, such as academic performance in school. Even if harm reduction is a short-term objective, most interventions try to move the individual toward the goal of abstinence. Other common goals or strategies across treatments include providing detailed information regarding the physical and psychological effects of drug use; working to shift the student's thoughts and beliefs so that the consequences of drug use are understood; and reducing the impact of *risk factors* (i.e., situations or characteristics that lead to increased drug use) while increasing the positive impact of *protective factors* (i.e., situation or characteristics that are associated with choosing not to use drugs: see Chapter 2 for a detailed discussion of risk and protective factors). For example, most interventions try to improve an adolescent's social relationships and social skills to some degree—perhaps by exploring the impact of peer relationships on drug use, recommending group therapy to build peer support and skills, or directly involving family members in the intervention. Finally, most interventions seek to improve the student's ability to cope with emotions and situations that result in the urge to use drugs, and to build skills for making healthy behavior choices (AACAP, 2005).

Although intervention programs share these general goals, in actual practice these adolescents are treated in many different ways.

Adolescents Are Treated in a Variety of Settings

If one of your students is facing serious drug use or your school does not have the resources needed to intervene directly, you may find yourself wanting to make a referral to a treatment program. Students and their parents may have questions about different treatment options. As a school mental health professional, you may be asked to work with the student's treatment team during and after intervention, and as the student returns to his or her school and home. Therefore, it will be helpful to understand the types of treatment settings that are typically available for adolescent drug use.

RESIDENTIAL AND INPATIENT SETTINGS

The most intensive and structured treatment settings are inpatient/hospital-based and residential (non-hospital-based) treatment programs. These treatments are usually reserved for students with severe addictions, or those students with substance problems and serious psychiatric symptoms (e.g., suicidality, violence). Inpatient programs are typically locked facilities (e.g., hospitals), with 24-hour supervision and structured schedules. Some adolescents may be there against their will, as several states allow parents to "voluntarily" commit their children. The amount of time an adolescent spends in residential or inpatient treatment typically ranges from about 1 week to 3 months, with an average of about 1 month for residential treatment and shorter stays in inpatient hospitals (Rutherford & Banta-Green, 1998). Due to changes in health insurance benefits, often adolescents stay just long enough to be assessed, to address the most serious problems, and to begin treatment that is continued in less restrictive and expensive settings (e.g., day treatment or outpatient therapy).

Treatment typically begins with a comprehensive assessment involving a multidisciplinary team, including physicians, nurses, psychiatrists, psychologists or counselors, social workers or case managers, and educational and residential staff. Particular attention is paid to assessing and treating any co-occurring mental health conditions, such as depression, suicidality, ADHD, or conduct problems, and sometimes medication is prescribed. The initial part of treatment sometimes involves a "blackout" period, where the adolescent is kept relatively isolated from other adolescent patients and family in order to allow detoxification or withdrawal symptoms to diminish. Most programs include individual therapy with a counselor, ranging from daily sessions to a few sessions a week. Adolescents attend daily group sessions, which focus on such topics as developing more healthy coping skills, improving peer and family relationships, and relapse prevention planning.

In many programs, family members are invited to become involved in treatment. Another typical feature is that staff members are trained to provide immediate feedback to the student aimed at identifying and altering problematic patterns of thinking and behavior choices. The student typically attends some sort of on-site educational program as well; this program may include having the adolescent complete schoolwork gathered from his or her school, or work on assignments related to substance use. Some educational programs conduct testing to assess for learning problems.

As the student gets ready to leave, the team makes recommendations for *aftercare*. Aftercare involves helping the adolescent and his or her family become involved in intervention services in their community, so that treatment can continue and the adolescent is supported as he or she returns home and school. Some treatment settings may have a "transitional program" designed to ease the adolescent back into independent life. In these programs, adolescents are gradually returned to the "natural environment"—either by returning home but attending *day treatment* or *partial hospitalization* (i.e., spending their days at the treatment facility), or by living in a monitored group home while returning to their regular community school (Rutherford & Banta-Green, 1998).

OUTPATIENT SETTINGS

Outpatient treatment, typically conducted at community mental health clinics, is the most commonly utilized approach for adolescent substance use. This setting is appropriate for most adolescents who are not experiencing physical dependence on substances or serious co-occurring psychiatric disorders (e.g., depression). Outpatient treatment offers the adolescent and family structured intervention, while allowing the adolescent to practice new skills or behavior changes in the "real" home and community environment. Such treatment varies in length, treatment orientation, and access to therapists trained in adolescent substance use intervention. In urban areas, it is possible to find community mental health agencies that offer some types of specific adolescent drug use intervention services. In more rural environments, there are fewer outpatient clinics or mental health professionals who are specially trained in adolescent substance use. Outpatient programs also vary greatly in intensity: Students in outpatient treatment may simply meet with a therapist once a week, or may attend an after-school treatment program every day with weekly family and individual therapy sessions. On average, the duration of outpatient treatment ranges from 3 to 6 months. Outpatient therapy can be a stand-alone treatment, but it is often also recommended as part of any aftercare plan when a student is returning home after inpatient or residential treatment (Rutherford & Banta-Green, 1998).

SCHOOL SETTINGS

By this point our readers may be thinking, "What are the individual interventions designed for school settings?" Given that a teacher or school mental health professional is sometimes the first to identify or recognize a student's problems with drugs, and that school personnel have daily contact with students, doesn't it make perfect sense to provide substance use interventions in schools? Well, as stated earlier, relatively few well-tested intervention programs for student substance use have been specifically developed for school personnel to conduct (Rones & Hoagwood, 2000; Wagner, Brown, Monti, Myers, & Waldron, 1999). Most individual interventions are designed for outpatient settings. Many intervention programs recognize the importance of involving teachers or counselors as part of the treatment team when students are being treated for substance abuse; however, involvement is usually defined by having school personnel monitor and provide information about student academic performance and behavior, rather than provide direct intervention. The lack of school-based individual interventions may seem surprising because of the many innovative and effective prevention programs that are currently conducted in schools nationwide (see Chapter 4 for a more detailed discussion of school-based prevention programs). Some such programs offer brief individual or group interventions, such as social skills groups, when students are identified as at high risk for drug use or as already having substance use problems. However, the developers of most of the large-scale prevention programs suggest referring students with more serious substance use behaviors to other treatment settings (e.g., outpatient or inpatient/residential programs).

One individual intervention model that has shown success in the school setting is known as the *student assistance program* (SAP) model (Gonet, 1994). To establish an SAP, school systems hire a certified counselor, or a counseling team, with special training in adolescent drug use assessment and treatment. Teachers, students, or others can anonymously refer a student to the SAP counselor. One goal of the SAP is to create an environment in which students and school professionals feel safe in raising potential drug use problems without fear of any retribution from peers or others. The SAP counselor investigates and assesses the referral with discretion and confidentiality. The SAP counselor may then conduct individual or group intervention, or refer the student and family to another setting, depending upon the severity of the problem. Many school districts have similar programs or groups of counselors, sometimes called a *faculty intervention team*, a *chemical assessment referral and education team*, or *intervention specialists* (Gonet, 1994). Although SAPs are available in some schools, a recent survey of school-based mental health services found that 43% of schools offered substance use counseling, and only 12% had a specified substance use counselor (Foster et al., 2005). At present, it is unclear how many students seek out or are referred to any school-based services, or receive individual counseling for drug use problems in schools nationwide (Rones & Hoagwood, 2000).

Adolescent Intervention Programs Reflect a Variety of Treatment Orientations

Treatment approaches differ depending upon underlying theories about how drugs affect an individual, how addiction processes occur, and how best to treat drug problems. Treatment orientations are roughly divided into four types, although there is typically significant overlap, as mental health professionals often "mix and match" strategies from different orientations to meet an individual adolescent's needs.

One orientation, referred to as the *Minnesota model* (Williams & Chang, 2000) or *12-step model*, is based on the idea that substance abuse or dependence is a chronic disease that must be recognized as a problem out of the student's control (Deas & Thomas, 2001). The intervention associated with this model involves a combination of individual and group therapy. Treatment usually starts with a brief stay (4–6 weeks) at a hospital or residential program, with outpatient therapy and attendance at Alcoholics/Narcotics Anonymous or similar groups. In this model, the power to change is gained from moving through "steps," in which the adolescent addresses denial, commits to abstinence, and chooses a healthy lifestyle. Changes are maintained through the supportive, reinforcing environment of group therapy with others recovering from substance use (see Chapter 6 for a detailed discussion of group interventions). Although this is a popular model designed for adults who use substances, it has only recently been tried with adolescents, and it is unclear how effective it is in reducing or eliminating adolescent drug use over the long term (Muck et al., 2001).

Cognitive-behavioral therapy (CBT) and *behavioral therapy* are also common orientations in inpatient and outpatient interventions. In these orientations, substance use is seen as a *learned behavior.* This means that an adolescent first learns to use drugs by seeing others do it (this is called *modeling*), and continues to use drugs because doing so produces *reinforcement* (either some type of reward or positive consequence, or a reduction or avoidance of negative consequences). The rewards may include the "positive rush" that comes with using some drugs, or the praise and admiration of friends, or the temporary experience of "lifting one's cares away" when the adolescent is feeling stressed or anxious. Over time, the adolescent begins to anticipate these reinforced responses automatically when he or she is in situations similar to the ones in which the adolescent has used drugs before. Just thinking about the situation, experiencing anxious thoughts or feelings, or being with particular friends becomes a cue to the adolescent that if he or she uses drugs, the temporary reward will ensue. In this way, a circular pattern of thoughts, feelings, and environmental cues leads to continued drug use. Interventions from a CBT or behavioral orientation focus on teaching a student to become aware of the connections among thoughts, beliefs, motivations, and environmental cues that are associated with wanting to use drugs. Essentially, the goal is to help the student decrease the substance-using behaviors and replace them with more positive behaviors and coping strategies that are incompatible with drug use. Mental health professionals help adolescents to identify and use better problem-solving and drug refusal skills, and to develop more positive ways to cope with strong emotions (e.g., using relaxation strategies). Other treatment strategies include helping the adolescent to learn how to resist peer pressure; to develop more positive peer and adult role models; and to become involved in positive, structured activities. One potent CBT strategy is *functional assessment*, in which the student is asked to identify the events that occurred right before the student decided to use the substance (e.g., "What happened right before you decided to drink? How were you feeling?"), how the student reacted (e.g., "How much did you drink?"), and consequences (e.g., "What happened next? What were the results of drinking?"). Functional assessment is used to help adolescents become aware of the situations in which they are at risk for drug use, gain insight into why they choose to use drugs, and to learn other action they can take that will lead to healthier outcomes. Later in this chapter, we present a sample functional assessment and a blank form to use with students in conducting such assessments. The CBT counselor also frequently teaches skills directly, and directs students to practice skills through homework and role-playing exercises. Sometimes the counselor will also develop a *behavior contract* with an adolescent; this is a written agreement that if the adolescent follows specific rules or steps to reduce substance use, he or she will receive a tangible reward, such as a desired item or free time (Monti, Abrams, Kadden, & Cooney, 1989).

Family-based treatments evolve from the idea that an adolescent's family members and relationships play a critical role in the development and maintenance of his or her drug use. Student drug use levels have been shown to be related to low-quality parent–adolescent relationships, problems in parent monitoring and parent–adolescent communication, substance use patterns of family members, and other family risks (Dishion & Kavanagh, 2003). From a family systems point of view, the student's drug use is a reflection of problems that are occurring at the family level; that is, the drug use is a "symptom" of a dysfunctional family system, and thus the entire family should be involved in treatment. In family systems counseling or therapy, the mental health professional typically observes interactions between family members and offers specific feedback to point out negative communication patterns and to clarify family members' roles and appropriate structure (e.g., "Parents are in charge"). Family therapists also try to "relabel" the problem (i.e., to discuss the adolescent's behavior from a different and potentially more positive perspective), in order to shift the family system toward taking some collective responsibility for the problem and solution (Austin, Macgowan, & Wagner, 2005). Other family-based treatments look at how to improve parental functioning and family relationships, in tandem with working on the student's substance use. For example, some programs offer weekly parenting groups that focus on teaching parents more effective ways to manage their adolescent's behavior through the use of positive reinforcement, to monitor their adolescent's activities, and to communicate more effectively with their adolescents (Dishion & Kavanagh, 2003; Kazdin, 2005). These *parent management training* programs are typically highly structured, with steps for the mental health professional to follow during each session, and practice materials for the parents to use. Increasingly, family-based treatments are used in conjunction with other individual treatments (such as behavioral therapy), with promising results (Dishion & Kavanagh, 2003; Waldron, Brody, & Slesnick, 2001).

A newer approach to working with drug-using adolescents is called *motivational enhancement therapy* (MET; Miller, Zweben, DiClemente, & Rychtarik, 1994). MET involves specific interviewing, assessment, and counselor feedback strategies designed to help adolescents increase motivation to change their behavior. From an MET perspective, it is assumed that most adolescents who use substances experience *ambivalence* about making a change in their drug use habits. That is, an adolescent may recognize the negative aspects of drug-using behavior, but may be discouraged by past failures to quit or resistant to change due to fears about what life would be like without the drug. The adolescent may also identify positive aspects to using drugs, such as acceptance among a particular peer group. Studies have shown that if a mental health professional can help an individual see the negative aspects of using drugs as more personally salient and distressing than the perceived rewards associated with the positive aspects, the individual will become more motivated to change the behavior (Prochaska & DiClemente, 1984). In

MET, this is called "tipping the decisional balance" toward positive change, and it is an important part of the intervention model. The MET counselor calls upon other motivational interviewing techniques (Miller & Rollnick, 1991, 2002), such as expressing empathy and reducing the adolescent's resistance to change by affirming the adolescent's abilities to make small changes (improving *self-efficacy*) and to build toward more lasting harm reduction or abstinence. Because MET techniques have been successfully tested in brief interventions with adults (sometimes demonstrating positive outcomes in one or two sessions!) and are well suited for resistant at-risk adolescents, MET components are currently being tested in research studies with both adolescents and adults; MET is combined in these studies with existing treatment methods, such as CBT, group therapy, or family treatment (Dishion & Kavanagh, 2003; Sampl & Kadden, 2000).

Pharmacotherapy, or intervening by prescribing medication to treat substance abuse, is infrequently used with adolescents unless addiction is severe, other treatments have failed, or serious co-occurring mental health problems are present. Prescribing medication for substance abuse in adolescents is rarely used as a stand-alone treatment (AACAP, 2005). The medications prescribed to adolescents are those typically used to treat adults with drug abuse, including methadone as a nonaddictive replacement for opioid addiction or naltrexone for alcohol dependence. Little research has evaluated the effectiveness of these drugs in treating adolescent drug use. More often, medications are prescribed for substance-using adolescents to treat co-occurring mental health conditions, such as mood disorders. For example, treatment with lithium during the manic phases of adolescent bipolar disorder appears to reduce drug use as well (Geller, 1998). Other research suggests that treating co-occurring depression with medications in the selective serotonin reuptake inhibitor class (e.g., Zoloft or Paxil), or the so-called "atypical antidepressant" class (e.g., Wellbutrin), is associated with reductions in drug use. Psychiatric medication that successfully treats the underlying mental health condition may lead to reductions in drug use because an adolescent could be using substances to manage or suppress symptoms, or to cope with strong negative emotions such as sadness and anxiety (Riggs, 2003). However, physicians must be cautious and monitor these students closely, as using illicit drugs increases potential of overdose, and some psychiatric medications can be addicting (AACAP, 2005).

Effectiveness of Current Interventions

Now that we have described many different individual interventions for substance use and abuse, our readers might be wondering, "What is the most effective treatment strategy?" Unfortunately, there is no easy answer to this question. The good news is that some treatment is better than no treatment (Catalano, Hawkins, Wells, & Miller, 1990; Deas & Thomas, 2001). This means that regardless of the type of treatment setting or orientation, adolescents who receive some sort of intervention for drug use demonstrate better outcomes (e.g., reduced drug use, lower rates of criminal involvement, higher grades in school, and improved psychological adjustment) than similar adolescents who do not receive any treatment (Dennis et al., 2004; Williams & Chang, 2000). Many different treatment approaches demonstrate positive changes in adolescent substance use; for instance, both inpatient and outpatient programs generally show positive short-term outcomes. However, there are no data available documenting the effectiveness of interventions conducted by school mental health professionals. Some studies suggest that schools with SAPs report lower student rates of alcohol use and higher academic achievement (Scott, Surface, Friedli, & Barlow, 1999; see also the website for Project Success, *www.sascorp.org*).

When alternative treatment approaches are compared with one another (rather than with a no-treatment group), programs that focus on the family (e.g., family therapy or parent management training) and those that combine family and individual interventions generally show better success than those interventions involving only an individual adolescent. Two such interventions are *integrated behavioral and family therapy* (Waldron et al., 2001) and the family-centered approach used in the Adolescent Transitions Program (ATP; Dishion & Kavanagh, 2003), which combine direct parent and adolescent skills training with family-focused therapy to improve communication and the quality of the relationships among family members. Another intervention, *functional family therapy* (Sexton & Alexander, 2000), targets family-level behaviors in treatment. These interventions demonstrate better long-term outcomes in many areas, including lower levels of substance use and better relationships with school, family members, and peers (Austin et al., 2005; Liddle, 2004). In a large multisite investigation that compared three different treatment components (i.e., short-term MET, CBT, and family treatment) for adolescent marijuana use, all three interventions produced significant reductions in drug use and other risks (such as involvement with drug-using peers), even at 3 and 12 months after the intervention ended (Dennis et al., 2004). Overall, the research suggests that although treatment works, no one intervention type has demonstrated consistent long-term decreases in adolescent substance use that are far superior to others (Rutherford & Banta-Green, 1998). Sufficient evidence does not exist to show which interventions work best for whom and under what conditions (Austin et al., 2005). We do know that once students complete treatment successfully, variables predicting long-term success include social support from family and peers, compliance with treatment plan, and continued motivation to reduce or quit drug use (AACAP, 2005; Brown, 2001).

Despite the promising results from studies that evaluate adolescent drug use interventions, relapse rates remain high. For example, one review reported that up to 60–70% of adolescents relapse 3–6 months following treatment (Rutherford & Banta-Green, 1998). The risk is highest during the first 3 months after treatment ends. These findings underscore the difficulties that students who have undergone treatment for substance use face in maintaining positive changes in their behavior. These statistics also highlight the critical need for identifying ways to support students after the intensive phase of the intervention has ended. For adolescents to continue the positive gains they have made in treatment, it is has been recommended that interventions include significant resources for long-term aftercare services (AACAP, 2005). Research has shown that adolescents who participate in intensive aftercare services have better long-term outcomes (Godley, Godley, & Dennis, 2001; Williams & Chang, 2000). Aftercare services that are especially promising include continued contact with a therapist, participation in community programs such as after-school recreation programs, and participation in support groups (Godley et al., 2001). However, having an identified *case manager*—that is, a person who is knowledgeable about the adolescent's and family's history, as well as the risks and resources that are available in the adolescent's environment—is also an essential part of successful aftercare intervention (Williams & Chang, 2000). The case manager's objective is to coordinate and assist in the implementation of a long-term plan to ensure that the student and family have the support they need to maintain treatment gains.

IMPORTANT QUESTIONS ABOUT INDIVIDUAL INTERVENTIONS FOR STUDENTS

What Are the Essential Components of Student Interventions?

Based on research and expert opinion, AACAP (2005) and CSAT (1999c) recommend that student treatment programs should include components to target the following:

- Motivation and engagement in making behavioral changes.
- Family involvement to improve supervision, monitoring, and communication.
- Development of skills to improve problem solving and behavior choices, and to prevent relapse.
- Co-occurring mental health disorders (through psychological or medication treatments).
- The social environment (prosocial behaviors, peer relationships, and academic functioning).
- Comprehensive aftercare planning.

Given the complex nature of adolescent substance use, it is not surprising that the recommended treatment involves multiple domains. Our readers may be looking at this list and thinking, "I don't have the resources, the time, or the energy to put together a comprehensive intervention like this, especially for one student!" It certainly may seem daunting to think about providing intervention at this level. Yet there may be areas in which schools and school professionals have the necessary intervention tools and resources to address these problems.

When Should a School Mental Health Professional Decide to Implement an Individual Intervention Plan?

Our second question is difficult to answer in brief, and it largely depends on what professionals and their schools are ready and willing to offer. There are different approaches to thinking about the school mental health professional's role and the appropriateness of conducting more intensive intervention. Because the recommendations listed above dictate that interventions should involve multiple components, some note that a school mental health professional should not be the primary intervention agent, and suggest that the role of the school is to provide support rather than to conduct individual interventions (Gonet, 1994). For example, many school counselors do not feel adequately trained to provide services to substance-using students (Burrow-Sanchez & Lopez, in press). It is certainly the case that for adolescents with serious substance use disorders, individual treatment is likely to require intensive treatment led by specialists (AACAP, 2005). However, when a student demonstrates less serious drug use (i.e., experimental or regular use without physical dependence), it is appropriate for a school mental health professional to consider administering an intervention, provided that the professional has adequate training, resources, and supervision (AACAP, 2005). The challenge is in assessing the level of adolescent substance use and risk and protective factors, and in distinguishing between those students who could benefit from an early intervention program and those who need greater levels of service (Gonet, 1994). This is why a comprehensive assessment of a student's substance use is always indicated as a first step (see Chapter 3 and "Pretreatment Assessment," below). In Figure 5.1, we offer some guidelines to assist you in making referral decisions (see also Chapter 7 for more specific information on the referral process).

What Is the School Professional's Role When the Student Is Receiving Treatment from an Outside Agency?

As mentioned above, most formal treatment for adolescent substance use occurs outside the school setting. This does not mean, however, that school personnel are not or should not be involved in the treatment process. School personnel may support or enhance treatment efforts in many ways. Their role in working with students, families, and treatment programs will vary according to the stage of treatment, the orientation of a particular program, its openness to involving school professionals, and other factors. Before communicating with treatment agencies, however, professionals must be sure to discuss their intentions regarding sharing of information and confidentiality parameters with adolescents and parents, and obtain signed consent to exchange information. Some of the roles that you may play as a school mental health professional in the intervention process include the following:

- *Providing home-bound instruction or information related to the student's educational and behavioral history.* Often the treatment agency will request copies of the student's school records (test scores, grades, disciplinary infractions, etc.) and any information pertaining to the student's substance use. Because many of these students have learning difficulties or demonstrate poor academic performance, treatment teams will sometimes request formal psychological and educational testing. You may be requested to conduct testing while a student is in treatment, or to develop an individualized education plan (IEP). Your knowledge about the student's school history, and about resources and accommodations available in your school district, will be extremely important in developing appropriate IEP goals and a comprehensive long-term plan.

Level of substance use and other risks

Experimental use
- Student is considering using or has just begun to use tobacco, alcohol, or drugs
- Student uses infrequently with friends

Regular use
- Student uses substances on an occasional but regular basis; may be expressed as significant binge drinking or drug use in social situations
- Low-level associated risk factors may be present (e.g., grades slipping, peer problems)

Problem use
- Student has experienced adverse consequences
- Student may demonstrate significant problems with grades, detentions, or suspensions; parent and peer relationships; injuries or motor vehicle accidents; or physical or sexual assaults

Substance abuse
- Student engages in ongoing use of drugs or alcohol, despite harm or significant risky behaviors or events ("close calls")
- Student reports loss of control over use
- Substance use patterns have led to problems in multiple domains of functioning (e.g., academic failure, deviant peer group)

Substance dependence
- Student is using frequently, despite clear risk of harm and dependence
- Student shows tolerance or symptoms of withdrawal
- Student demonstrates significant and increasing risk-taking and dangerous drug-related behaviors
- Substance use patterns have led to problems in multiple domains of functioning (e.g., school, home, work, relationships)
- Student's own attempt to stop using substances have failed repeatedly

Suggested level of intervention

Brief school-based counseling
- Education about risks and consequences
- Explore options for change

School-based counseling
- Build motivation for change
- Development of coping skills
- Family involvement if appropriate

Outpatient therapy referral
- Particularly if you have concerns about comorbid conditions or significant family stress

Intensive outpatient therapy
Integrated outpatient/family therapy

Partial or day treatment program

Residential treatment

Inpatient treatment

FIGURE 5.1. Guidelines for matching student needs with intervention settings. Arrows indicate appropriate levels of intervention and movement between intervention types.

- *Serving as a liaison among the treatment agency, school, and family.* This may require attending interagency team meetings to provide consultation on an educational and transition plan. Sometimes adolescents and their families have developed negative relationships with their schools' administrators, because of repeated disciplinary infractions or behavior problems have left school members exasperated and unwilling to give the students another chance. In such a case, you may need to help bridge the communication barriers between family and school to develop an appropriate long-term education plan. Your role also could include informing other school personnel who need to know about the treatment and relapse prevention plan (e.g., teachers, coaches), although it is critical to preserve confidentiality whenever possible (see Chapter 1 for a more detailed discussion of confidentiality).

- *Being an advocate for the student's educational needs during treatment.* Many states mandate that students in residential treatment receive some educational instruction, but not all treatment programs have the resources to provide teachers or well-trained teaching staff, or may not utilize this time to improve a student's academic performance. Also, many students have fallen behind because of frequent absences or interference from substance use. You may be asked to supply educational materials so that a student does not fall further behind. It may be possible to arrange for the student to receive academic credit for any classwork (e.g., attending classes on harm reduction) completed as part of the intervention. You may have to be creative with planning to meet the specific needs of the student.

- *Working with the treatment team, adolescent, and family to develop a comprehensive plan for reintegration into school, and monitoring implementation of the plan.* Transition planning is a critical component for success, and you can play a leadership role in this planning. Here are some suggested steps to consider:

  - Set clear expectations and consequences for the student's behavior upon returning to school.
  - Develop a relapse prevention plan and understand your potential role (e.g., part of the plan may be to have the student come see you if he or she is feeling stressed).
  - Identify the key treatment team members and their roles, and obtain contact information for follow-up questions and concerns.
  - Assist the student and treatment team in anticipating situations in the school environment that may make the student vulnerable to relapse, so that the relapse plan is comprehensive and tailored to the student's context and the available resources.
  - Consider the student's academic placement—you may want to suggest a different placement when the student returns to school (i.e., alternative school, small-group classroom), or specific accommodations through a Section 504 plan.
  - Arrange a transition period in which the student initially spends part of the day in school, and part of the day in the treatment facility or home, with gradual increases until the student is in school full-time. Set up the student's schedule so that he or she is busy and under adult supervision whenever possible.

- Meet with the family and develop a communication plan for home–school continuity.
- If appropriate, arrange for a peer mentor in the school to provide extra support for the student.
- Help the adolescent and family to identify and enroll in positive, structured activities, so that the student's unstructured time is minimized and adult supervision is maximized.

We have noted earlier that *aftercare* is considered a key to successful treatment outcome (Muck et al., 2001). Unfortunately, many treatment agencies develop a detailed aftercare plan but provide no follow-up to ensure that the plan is successfully implemented. One potential role for a school mental health professional would be to serve in a coordinating or case management role with the adolescent and family in implementing the aftercare plan. The reality is that most schools do not have the resources to put toward this task. Schools should not take this on as a primary responsibility unless there are ample resources available. One guide that may be helpful is the Assertive Aftercare Protocol (also known as Assertive Continuing Care or ACC), a 12-session case management program for adolescent drug users who have been in inpatient or residential treatment (Godley et al., 2001). This program was developed for a treatment study, and the aftercare services were provided by mental health professionals in adolescents' homes, but the program manual contains materials that could easily be adapted for school personnel. ACC case managers focus on continuing the intervention by promoting prosocial behaviors and relapse prevention, but they also attend to such issues as reduction of barriers to engagement, crisis management, ongoing assessment of needs, and transportation. ACC case managers also target family motivation and provide education and teach skills to reduce risks for relapse. The ACC program is an intensive approach to aftercare, and it is not likely to be feasible for school personnel to implement the entire program. Again, however, ACC may be useful for school mental health professionals who are looking for guidance and materials to use with students to help reinforce skills learned in inpatient or residential treatment as the student returns to home and school.

Even if your role as a school professional does not include coordinating aftercare programming, you can support the process informally. One key role you *can* serve for students is being a source of support and encouragement. If the students see you as someone who will not judge them for behavior choices, the likelihood that they will seek out assistance when faced with vulnerability to a "slip" or relapse is much greater. It is important to make it clear to your students that your "door is always open."

A COMPREHENSIVE EARLY INTERVENTION PROGRAM

In this section, we offer a structured outline for school mental health professionals who are interested in conducting their own interventions with students demonstrating early or mild substance problems (see Table 5.1). In searching for an appropriate intervention,

TABLE 5.1. Suggested Structure for Intervention Based on MET and CBT

Session topics and goals	Intervention tasks and tools
Pretreatment assessment: • Comprehensive assessment for Personalized Feedback Report (PFR)	• (GAIN-Q Full) is administered • School mental health professional prepares PFR
Session 1: Build motivation • Build rapport and collaboration • Familiarize student with intervention • Begin assessing and building motivation to address substance use • Help student set initial goals	• School mental health professional uses MET techniques (e.g., express interest/empathy, provide nonjudgmental reactions) • Review PFR together (address ambivalence and develop discrepancies) • Give educational handout related to drug use • Summarize progress and any initial steps that the student has agreed to try
Session 2: Build motivation and goals • Continue to build motivation • Discuss potential benefits of action and likely negative consequences of inaction • Develop targets, goals, and steps for change	• Continue review of PFR, using cues from student to elicit ideas and potential plans for addressing drug use • Complete Decisional Balance Sheet (Figure 5.2) • Complete Change Plan Worksheet (Figure 5.3) • Summarize by highlighting progress, explicitly reviewing steps the student has agreed to try
Session 3: Strengthen commitment • Renew motivation and set goals • Introduce concept of functional assessment, and explore student's personal awareness of antecedents and consequences of drug use	• Discuss progress, thoughts, and reactions to intervention efforts • Re-review targets and goals, with positive reinforcement for change behavior • Complete the Knowledge Is Power Worksheet • Complete Personal Goals Worksheet
Sessions 4 and 5: Coping skills • Review functional assessment, and emphasize need to develop skills to cope with high-risk situations • Develop drug refusal skills	• Review importance of developing refusal skills • Refusal Skills handout • Complete Real Life Practice: Refusal Skills Worksheet
Sessions 6 and 7: Social support • Enhance social support network • Increase pleasurable activities	• Review Social Supports Reminder Sheet • Complete Social Circle Worksheet • Complete Real Life Practice: Seeking and Giving Support Worksheet
Sessions 8 and 9: Relapse prevention • Practice coping skills • Develop relapse prevention plan	• Discuss need for preparation for unanticipated high-risk relapse situations • List events that could precipitate a relapse • Introduce Steps for Problem Solving approach • Complete Personal Emergency Plan Worksheet

Note. Adapted from Sampl and Kadden (2000); in the public domain. All worksheets from Session 3 onward can be found in Sampl and Kadden.

we looked for the following characteristics: (1) It should be comprehensive, but ideally should not overburden busy school personnel; (2) it should be specifically designed to treat substance-using adolescents; (3) its strategies should have evidence supporting their success; (4) it should be appropriate to adapt for a school setting; and (5) it should offer clear instructions and obtainable materials. A decade ago, this search probably would have been futile. However, with the push for conducting sound intervention studies and the public dissemination of intervention materials, access to good treatment strategies is now readily available (AACAP, 2005; CSAT, 1999a, 1999b, 1999c).

The Basis for Our Intervention Program

The intervention structure we suggest below is primarily based on an intervention that was designed and tested in a large-scale research project, the Cannabis Youth Treatment (CYT) project series (Diamond et al., 2002). The CYT project developed and tested five different intervention protocols, and involved over 600 adolescent marijuana users from different sites across the country. This study was the first to create and compare intervention approaches for adolescent substance use on a large scale. The basic intervention combined the MET approach (two individual sessions with the adolescent) with three sessions of group-based CBT, for a total of five sessions (we call this the *brief adolescent-focused* intervention model). The MET and CBT approaches were adapted specifically for adolescents, drawing from similar intervention strategies tested with adults (Kadden et al., 1995; Monti et al., 1989; Steinberg, Carroll, Roffman, & Kadden, 1997). One of the other interventions tested in the study consisted of the same intervention with seven group-based CBT sessions added (we call the *longer adolescent-focused* model). The third intervention combined the longer adolescent-focused model with the Family Support Network, an additional intervention involving four home sessions with the families and six parent group education sessions. In a second study, two other types of family interventions were compared to the longer adolescent-focused intervention. The results indicated that all intervention types were effective in reducing marijuana use at 3- and 12-month follow-ups. However, in terms of cost-effectiveness, the two adolescent-focused interventions (brief and longer) were superior (Dennis et al., 2004).

Each of these CYT interventions was designed for the treatment of adolescents ages 12–18 who use marijuana. However, the authors note that the treatment strategies are similar to those that are effective for other types of problems (e.g., alcohol, smoking), and that the materials they used in sessions are suitable for treating other substances. They caution that adolescents who use multiple drugs (e.g., alcohol, marijuana, and methamphetamines), who need a higher level of care than outpatient therapy, or who have other serious mental health disorders should be referred to a more intensive treatment (see Figure 5.1). The authors indicate that an adolescent-focused program is likely to be well suited for early intervention in a school setting when conducted by experienced school mental health professionals. There are several excellent sources of information available to guide school mental health professionals in conducting intervention sessions; we list these at the end of this chapter (see "Chapter Resources").

It is important to note that the session order and content of sessions are flexible, and that school mental health professionals can easily tailor topics or techniques to the particular needs of the student, or draw upon additional materials from other intervention programs. We urge our readers to explore other materials (again, see the "Chapter Resources" section) and experiment to find the techniques that work for them and for their schools. For example, many of the prevention programs designed for school settings (see Chapter 4) have well-developed materials and media resources that could also be easily used during one-to-one counseling or social skills training sessions.

A Brief Adolescent-Focused, School-Based Intervention for Substance Use

Our adaptation of the CYT project's brief adolescent-focused intervention involves three phases or components that are implemented consecutively: (1) a comprehensive pre-intervention structured assessment; (2) initial sessions utilizing MET techniques to build engagement and help the student become committed to making positive changes; and (3) CBT-based sessions that focus on developing coping and relapse prevention skills. Table 5.1 lists the suggested sequence for the sessions. The session topics closely follow the descriptions in the original CYT intervention manual (Sampl & Kadden, 2000), except that we have suggested spreading the session goals and activities across more sessions, due to probable time constraints when conducted in a school setting. The original CBT-based sessions were administered in a group format, but the techniques, materials, and instructions are all appropriate for use in individual counseling sessions.

The steps and techniques used in the first few sessions are based primarily on MET. However, school mental health professionals will probably find it useful to use motivational strategies throughout the intervention. We highly recommend that such professionals learn more about MET and motivational interviewing principles and techniques, as these strategies have shown great success in helping to break down the typical barriers between therapists and adolescent clients (Lambie, 2004). In our experience, motivational interviewing offers powerful tools to establish rapport, build trust, reduce arguments and power struggles, and minimize resistance to change in at-risk, highly resistant adolescents (see "Chapter Resources").

Pretreatment Assessment

Chapter 3 has described the critical importance of assessment prior to intervention. In the brief adolescent-focused approach, the pretreatment assessment involves the completion of a comprehensive protocol of psychological measures and interview. The results are used to prepare individualized feedback that offers a realistic and objective appraisal of the student's substance use patterns compared to those of the general population; identifies potentially negative contributors and consequences to substance use; and identifies potential motivators for change (Miller & Rollnick, 1991, 2002). The authors of the adolescent-focused interventions tested in the CYT suggest administering the Global Appraisal of Individual Needs (GAIN), a comprehensive evaluation suitable for determining a plan for brief interventions, screening and referrals, diagnosis, and treatment placement and planning (Dennis, Titus, White, & Hodgkins, 2002). There is a quick version (the GAIN-Q Full) that takes approximately 20–30 minutes to complete, and the student can complete it or school personnel can administer it. The GAIN-Q assesses the student's personal, family, and academic background; current sources of stress; physical, emotional, and behavioral health; other substance-related issues; and reasons for quitting drugs. Scores on the GAIN-Q Full will show how the adolescent's level of risk and protective factors and current drug use patterns compare to those of same-age peers—an important tool in helping the adolescent to realistically appraise the role drug use is playing in his or her life. These scores are used to generate a Personalized Feedback Report (PFR). The GAIN-Q Full is free and available in written and computerized formats (see the "Chapter Resources" section for information about obtaining the GAIN-Q Full and the PFR).

Sessions 1–3: Building and Strengthening Motivation to Change

The objectives of the initial sessions are to build a collaborative relationship between the school mental health professional and the student; to enhance the student's motivation to address his or her substance use; to introduce the concept of functional assessment; and to set some initial goals for change (Table 5.1). The manual for the brief adolescent-focused intervention from the CYT study (Sampl & Kadden, 2000) guides the school mental health professional through the tasks and techniques to be introduced in these sessions (see also other recommended resources), but below we elaborate upon a few key concepts. As stated earlier, *it is critical for the school mental health professional to interact with the student in a nonjudgmental manner, and allow the student to be open and honest about his or her drug use and decision-making processes.* This approach helps to establish rapport and trust. The philosophy underlying MET is that only the student can choose to make changes, and most substance-using adolescents will be ambivalent or resistant about this process. The adolescent is likely to see benefits in continuing the substance use (e.g., "My friends all do it; I don't want to be different from them") as well as benefits in changing (e.g., "If I stopped using drugs, I might do better in school"). Students will continue to use drugs if they perceive the benefits to outweigh the perceived negative consequences of changing their behavior. The decision to quit drug use occurs when a student perceives the benefits associated with making changes in drug use to be more important than the benefits of continued use. This type of reasoning is called *decisional balance.* The objective in the initial intervention sessions is to attempt to shift this balance from the status quo (i.e., continued drug use) toward making changes (i.e., reduced drug use or abstinence; Miller et al., 1999).

There are several practical strategies for building motivation and tipping the balance toward making positive changes, most of which involve motivational interviewing (Miller & Rollnick, 1991, 2002). A few strategies based on those in the brief adolescent-focused intervention manual are described below to give you a sense of what this involves:

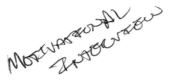

- *Eliciting self-motivational statements.* It is important that students find internal motivation and feel capable of making changes. The school mental health professional can help to increase this process by asking open-ended questions, such as "Tell me what you have noticed about your drug use. What concerns do you have or problems have you noticed as a result of using drugs?" Any concerns or ambivalent feelings raised by the student are used to help the student identify how the drug use may be having negative effects or getting in the way of achieving important goals, such as doing well in school. For example, "You aren't sure you want to stop drinking, but you recognize that it has led to some poor choices and problems in relationships, and you want better relationships in your life."

- *Listening and responding with empathy.* Adolescents will be resistant to adult directions and suggestions, especially when they perceive an adult as an adversary or as someone who will preach or moralize about their decision to use substances. A statement like "It is hard for you to imagine yourself living without alcohol" conveys an understanding of the student's perspective, and allows the student to be open to admitting any fears or ambivalent feelings about using drugs.

- *Supporting the student's steps to make changes.* Affirmations, or statements that acknowledge the student's ability to make changes, increase self-efficacy and reinforce positive steps. An example is "You really have come up with some great places to start to make changes."

- *Handling resistance.* There are a number of ways to reduce resistance, including "rolling with it." This is used to keep the conversation moving forward when students show extreme opposition. This can be seen in the following exchange:

STUDENT: I can't quit drinking because that is what me and my friends do!

COUNSELOR: Sounds like you don't want to stop drinking because it's something you can do with your friends?

STUDENT: Yeah.

COUNSELOR: Tell me more about drinking with your friends.

These strategies and others are used when the school mental health professional reviews the PFR with the student during the first few sessions. The feedback is used as a starting point for identifying and elaborating the "pros and cons" involved in choosing to continue drug use. The PFR is also used to point out inaccurate perceptions about drug use (e.g., "Everyone your age isn't also drinking every weekend. In fact, it looks like you are drinking more than 85% of other girls your age"). The school mental health professional also highlights the potential benefits of quitting or reducing drug use, using the student's own responses to make these salient to the student. Other steps in these early sessions include completing the Decisional Balance Worksheet (see Figure 5.2), Change Plan Worksheet (see Figure 5.3), Personal Goal Worksheet (see Figure 5.4), and Functional Assessment Worksheet (see Figure 5.5). The aim of these exercises is to set some

In making a decision to change, it can be helpful to think about the **good things** and **less good things** about using alcohol and/or drugs.

Below, write in the reasons you can think of in each of the boxes. For most people, "making a change" will probably mean quitting alcohol and drugs, but it is important that you consider what specific change you might want to make, which may be something else.

Good things about using	**Less good things about using**
Less good things about reducing or stopping	**Good things about reducing or stopping**

FIGURE 5.2. Decisional Balance Worksheet.

The changes I want to make are:

The most important reasons why I want to make these changes are:

The steps I plan to take in changing are:

The ways other people can help me are:
Person   Possible ways to help

I will know that my plan is working if:

Some things that could interfere with my plan are:

FIGURE 5.3. Change Plan Worksheet.

This is my goal regarding my drug use:

_____
_____
_____
_____
_____

Here are some important reasons for my goal:

_____
_____
_____
_____
_____
_____
_____
_____
_____
_____

The steps I plan to take to achieve my goal are:

_____
_____
_____
_____
_____
_____
_____
_____
_____
_____
_____

Name _____   Date _____

FIGURE 5.4. Personal Goal Worksheet.

Introduction: When we think about substance use, we often think about it as a negative habit. We think that substance use doesn't just happen, however. Usually there are things that are going on in a person's life or in the way they are thinking or feeling that affects whether a person decides to use substances. Knowing what affects your own use gives you more power to decide whether or not to use substances. We are going to use this sheet to figure out some of the factors that lead to your substance use. The idea is to show the many different ways in which you can break the habit, and take back control instead of being under control of the habit.

Personal Awareness: What Happens before and after I Use Substances?

Trigger	Thoughts and feelings	Behavior	Positive results	Negative results
(What sets me up to be more likely to use substances?)	(What was I thinking? What was I feeling? What did I tell myself?)	(What did I do then?)	(What good things happened?)	(What bad things happened?)

FIGURE 5.5. Functional Assessment Worksheet.

initial goals and assist the student in figuring out how to go about taking steps toward those goals. At the beginning of every session, progress toward goals is reviewed, and any positive changes made by the student are praised. If no progress was made, the student and school mental health professional focus on renewing commitment to make the change. As guides for the school mental health professional, Figures 5.6 and 5.7 include comments in italics for the Decisional Balance Worksheet and the Change Plan Worksheet, respectively.

In making a decision to change, it can be helpful to think about the good things and less good things about using alcohol and/or drugs.

Below, write in the reasons you can think of in each of the boxes. For most people, "making a change" will probably mean quitting alcohol and drugs, but it is important that you consider what specific change you might want to make, which may be something else.

Good things about using	**Less good things about using**
Examples of positive results of the behavior might include:	*Examples of negative results of the behavior might include:*
I don't have to deal with my problems *I feel more confident* *I have something to do when I am bored* *I use to fit in with my friends* *I have more fun at parties* *It helps me calm down and relax*	*I feel guilty or ashamed* *I don't like the way I look and feel after use* *It is a source of conflict between me and my family* *It is a source of conflict between me and my friends* *I will have money problems* *I will continue to feel anxious and depressed* *I will harm my health*
Less good things about reducing or stopping	**Good things about reducing or stopping**
Examples of negative results of changing the behavior might include:	*Examples of positive results of changing the behavior might include:*
I will feel more depressed and/or anxious *I won't have anything to do when I'm bored* *I won't have any way to relax* *I will have to change my social life* *I won't fit in with some friends* *I don't know if I can make change stick*	*I will feel more in control over my life* *I will gain more self-esteem* *It will improve my relationship with my family* *I will have more money* *I will have fewer problems at school and/or work* *It will make it easier to achieve life goals*

FIGURE 5.6. Decisional Balance Worksheet, with guidelines for the school mental health professional. Comments in italics are presented as guides for the school mental health professional. From Sobell and Sobell (1993). Copyright 1993 by The Guilford Press. Adapted by permission.

The changes I want to make are:
- *In what ways or areas does the student want to make a change? Be specific.*
- *Include goals that are positive and active (e.g., beginning something, doing more of something), as well as the common goals of stopping, avoiding certain behaviors, etc.*

The most important reasons why I want to make these changes are:
- *What are the likely consequences of action and inaction?*
- *Which motivations for change seem most compelling to the student?*

The steps I plan to take in changing are:
- *How does the student plan to achieve these goals?*
- *How could the desired change be accomplished?*
- *Within the general plan and strategies described, what are some specific, concrete first steps that the student can take?*
- *When, where, and how will these steps be taken?*

The ways other people can help me are:

Person   Possible ways to help
- *In what ways could other people (e.g., parents, peers, siblings, other adults) help the student in taking these steps toward change?*
- *How will the student arrange for such support?*

I will know that my plan is working if:
- *What does the student hope will happen as a result of this change plan?*
- *What benefits could be expected from this change?*

Some things that could interfere with my plan are:
- *What situations or changes could undermine the plan?*
- *What else could go wrong?*
- *How could the student stick with the plan despite these problems or setbacks?*

FIGURE 5.7. Change Plan Worksheet, with guidelines for the school mental health professional. Comments in italics are presented as guides for the school mental health professional. Adapted from Miller, Zweben, DiClemente, and Rychtarik (1999); in the public domain.

Sessions 4–9: Developing and Practicing Skills for Maintaining Changes

The next several sessions are devoted to teaching and practicing skills that will help the student to maintain positive changes. The topics to discuss, the CBT-based exercises, and materials designed to help learn the skills are listed in Table 5.1. Because CBT approaches are likely to be more familiar to school mental health professionals than those based on MET, we review the goals and tasks of this phase of intervention more briefly. We refer school mental health professionals to the CYT adolescent-focused intervention manual (Sampl & Kadden, 2000) and to other resources listed at the end of the chapter, for more detailed information.

The primary objective of these sessions is to help students learn important coping skills that are associated with reducing drug use or maintaining abstinence. Thus the sessions center on identifying high-risk situations that may increase the likelihood of drug-using behavior, including external events (e.g., peers who use, stressful situations) and thoughts and feelings (e.g., urges, depressed mood). Students are also asked to practice strategies to cope with these high-risk situations, which will help the students to be more likely to apply the skills in "real life." The first two of these sessions (Sessions 4 and 5) center on ways to refuse to use drugs, including avoiding people who may exert pressure or trigger the desire to use, developing skills to handle any pressure to use, and practicing these skills so that they can be automatically recalled in the moment. The next two sessions (Sessions 6 and 7) address how to identify sources of support and how to ask for the types of support that a student may need to keep away from drugs. These sessions also involve identifying ways to increase the student's activities in environments that are supportive of non-drug-using behavior. The idea is to replace drug use behaviors with healthy behaviors. The final two sessions in the intervention (Sessions 8 and 9) involve working with the student to plan for moments when he or she may be vulnerable to falling back into drug use patterns (relapse prevention). The student and school mental health professional draw up a "personal emergency plan" and practice the plan. During this phase, the school mental health professional emphasizes that if the student does relapse or "slip," he or she has the ability and skills needed to make changes again (self-efficacy).

Additional Individual Sessions

At the end of the intervention, the hope is that the student is equipped with the motivation and commitment to reduce or abstain from drug use, and has learned how to make good decisions and maintain positive changes. However, there may be additional areas of concern that were not directly addressed in these sessions, or areas in which a student might benefit from more learning and practice. The longer adolescent-focused intervention manual used in the CYT study (Sampl & Kadden, 2000) outlines a number of additional session topics and materials for the sessions (Kadden et al., 1992; Monti et al., 1989; Webb, Scudder, Kaminer, & Kadden, 2002). These additional sessions address a variety of important topics, such as anger awareness, anger management, effective communication, coping with cravings and urges, depression management, and managing thoughts about drug use (Webb et al., 2002). For example, if a student reports depressive symptoms, a "Depression Management" session may be useful. In addition, we list other sources for "best-practices" combination prevention–intervention models in the "Chapter Resources" section. These programs also offer materials that may be useful for particular intervention targets.

Special Issues in Intervening with Substance-Using Students

Family Involvement

Family involvement in the intervention process is a recommended and effective component for long-term success (AACAP, 2005). For school personnel, it may be difficult or unrealistic to involve family members directly in the intervention process, beyond communicating about a student's performance and behavior in home and school settings. By the time the student's drug use comes to light, the parents may have been struggling with managing the student's behavior for a long time. They may feel frustrated and angry with their adolescent, and may seem unmotivated and resistant to addressing the problem at first. Parents may also feel a sense of blame and responsibility, which may lead them to act defensive when talking about what family factors may be affecting the student's drug use patterns. It is critical in work with families to use the same motivational principles described above. Parents often respond more positively to intervention efforts if they feel that school personnel understand the challenges they face; thus listening with empathy and expressing concern without making judgments about the parents are key strategies. Like adolescents, parents will need to feel supported and empowered to make changes. If you are interested in working as a school mental health professional with family members, the following intervention targets may be beneficial (based in part on Hamilton, Brantley, Tims, Angelovich, & McDougall, 2002):

- Provide education regarding typical adolescent development, family systems, and the development of drug abuse (e.g., tip sheets for parents from the National Clearinghouse for Alcohol and Drug Use Information [NCADI]; see "Chapter Resources").
- Help families identify treatment options in their community and connect to family support networks (e.g., Families Anonymous).
- Work with family members to identify ways to improve communication and increase positive activities.
- Improve parents' effectiveness in establishing appropriate authority, roles, rules, boundaries, routines, discipline, conflict resolution, and school–home communication.

As with students, the most important role you may play for families is as a source of support and information. It is beneficial to let family members know that you are available for consultation or support if and when they are ready to consider making changes. Sometimes when a student's drug problem comes to light, a family member's problem with drugs is also discovered. Therefore, it is important to be ready with information and support for a parent or sibling who may want to seek treatment as well.

Co-Occurring Mental Health Problems

As noted in Chapter 1, up to half of adolescents with serious substance use problems may also have co-occurring mental health conditions (AACAP, 2005). It is important to assess carefully for such problems prior to intervention. Common co-occurring conditions (such as conduct problems, ADHD, depression, or anxiety) can have a major impact on a student's engagement and motivation in treatment, or can increase the risk of relapse (Riggs, 2003). For example, if a student is primarily using drugs to alleviate underlying mood disturbances, a successful intervention will need to address the source and treat the mood issues concurrently. When other problems are present, the intervention should combine and integrate the best treatment techniques used to treat each problem—not just one or the other (Riggs & Davies, 2002). In many cases, this will involve a combination of medication and other interventions for mental health problems (e.g., CBT for anxiety). When the mental health condition is successfully treated, drug use is often reduced as well (Riggs, 2003). However, these students must be monitored carefully, because abuse potential exists with some medications and because some conditions (depression, conduct problems) may increase students' risky and harmful behaviors when they are also using drugs. Thus our recommendation is to refer students with these types of problems for further evaluation in an outpatient medical setting.

Cultural Issues in School-Based Interventions

There is some evidence that students of different ethnic and cultural backgrounds are exposed to different risk and protective factors associated with student substance use (Wallace & Muroff, 2002). As school mental health professionals, it is essential for us to be sensitive to potential cultural influences, but also not automatically assume that those influences affect drug use. Culturally based factors can help us understand differences and similarities in drug use patterns and the likelihood that adolescents and families will seek out intervention. For example, in one study, Asian American and Hispanic adolescents were consistently less likely to seek out treatment than non-Hispanic European American adolescents (Brown, 2001). Cultural factors can also be identified and enhanced as protective factors for reduced drug use. In a study of Hispanic adolescents, Marsiglia, Miles, Dustman, and Sills (2002) found that the strong emphasis on family cohesion and parental monitoring, investment in school, and commitment to religious activities often seen in this cultural group protected adolescents against drug use. The intervention program we have reviewed in this chapter was tested with multiethnic samples, and the manual's authors note that the activities are appropriate for different ethnic and cultural groups (Sampl & Kadden, 2000). We would recommend that school personnel learn more about the process of adapting intervention approaches to cultural groups. Resources for information regarding cultural issues can be found at the NCADI website and the school-based mental health center websites listed at the end of this chapter.

CASE EXAMPLE

Jack, a 14-year-old high school freshman, was doing poorly in school. His English teacher overheard him talking with classmates about events that involved binge-drinking episodes and risky behavior, including fighting. The teacher shared her concerns with the school psychologist, Mr. Tom Harder, who arranged to meet with Jack. Mr. Harder started by stating that he had heard some concerns about Jack's performance in school and potential problems with peers and drinking. Mr. Harder noted that while he hoped to discuss these concerns, this was also an opportunity for Jack to talk about any other experiences in his life. Understanding that Jack might be unwilling to talk openly without some ground rules, Mr. Harder first talked about confidentiality and the limits of confidentiality. After Jack consented to speak with him on these terms, Mr. Harder asked him, "Why don't we start with you telling me about what happened this last weekend, and how alcohol was involved?" Mr. Harder's intentions were to create a safe and nonjudgmental environment for Jack to talk openly, and to get Jack's perspective about these concerns, including his pattern of drinking. Mr. Harder employed motivational interviewing techniques to improve rapport. Jack acknowledged not meeting all of his responsibilities at school, but didn't see alcohol use as related to his school problems, because "I only drink on the weekends." Jack denied ever trying marijuana or other drugs. When Mr. Harder inquired whether Jack was aware of any problems related to his drinking, Jack admitted getting involved in fist fights at parties with "random guys." Jack also expressed concern about his new peer group, whose members had introduced him to drinking. He reported that he did not feel close to his new friends and that he missed playing basketball with his former peer group. Jack described feeling distracted, unmotivated, and bored in school as well. Mr. Harder asked Jack to consider possible links between the problems he was having and his alcohol use. Jack acknowledged that his heavy drinking had led to some poor choices, particularly the fighting. As a result of Mr. Harder's style of empathic responding, Jack began to talk about problems occurring at home. He described that his mother became angry when Jack came home late, especially if she noticed that he had been drinking. Jack also talked about how he and his mother fought "almost constantly" since his parents divorced several months ago. Jack said that at times, he thought his desire to drink heavily was in part to keep him from thinking about his family problems.

At the end of this discussion, Mr. Harder reflected that while Jack didn't see his drinking pattern as a direct problem related to his schoolwork, it seemed to him that "you may have some concerns about how the drinking has been affecting your relationships with friends and family." He went on to ask Jack whether he would be willing to fill out some questionnaires, and to meet again to review the information from them and talk more about these issues. They agreed that Mr. Harder would speak with Jack's mother about the concerns and this initial plan, and would gain her permission to continue meeting to address the concerns. They arranged to have Jack complete the GAIN-Q-Full. Before their next meeting, Mr. Harder scored the instrument and prepared a PFR.

At their next few weekly meetings, Mr. Harder and Jack reviewed the PFR. The PFR reflected that Jack's use of alcohol was much higher than that of other boys his age. Jack's responses also indicated a high level of family stress, mild symptoms of depression, and difficulty in managing anger. Jack was initially resistant to the fact that his pattern of drinking was more frequent and problematic than that of most boys his age. However, Jack reflected that the objective feedback helped him see how his drinking might be negatively affecting some important areas in his life. He agreed to work with Mr. Harder to identify some steps he could take to reduce his drinking. Mr. Harder and Jack then completed the Decisional Balance and Change Plan Worksheets. Jack first agreed to limit his drinking to one weekend night and to arrange to spend time playing basketball with his former peers on the other night. Jack was reluctant to set any goals related to his relationship with his mother, stating that "she doesn't care anyway," and Mr. Harder did not press the issue. At the next session, Jack reported that he had enjoyed his time playing basketball with his old friends, whereas the night spent drinking with his other friends had resulted in another "pointless fight." Mr. Harder praised Jack for following through on his plan, and noted Jack's phrasing of "pointless fight" to continue exploring the ways in which drinking and the new peer group might be leading Jack down a potentially negative path.

Mr. Harder then began to work with Jack on developing alcohol refusal skills and a plan for what to do when Jack perceived that he was at risk of drinking "too much" (Jack stated that his goal was to gain some control over the amount he was drinking, not to attain abstinence). Mr. Harder also decided to incorporate some sessions on anger awareness and management of anger and depression. Mr. Harder explored whether Jack would be willing to allow him to invite Jack's mother to attend a session, in order to talk about their patterns of communication and about "ways for them to be supportive of one another." Jack agreed, and a family session was planned. By this time, Jack was spending more time with his same-age, positive peer group and reported drinking only occasionally. Mr. Harder felt that Jack was on a more successful path, and was looking forward to continuing the intervention with Jack and getting his mother involved in the intervention.

CHAPTER SUMMARY

Our aims in this chapter have been to review the ways in which substance-using adolescents are currently treated, to introduce essential elements for delivering or supporting an effective individual intervention, and to provide guidance for implementing such an intervention in the school setting. School mental health professionals can play many roles in the assessment and intervention process, ranging from support and consultation to providing direct intervention services. Most students who are demonstrating significant problems with substance use are referred to outpatient or inpatient/residential treatment programs. There are few available structured treatments developed specifically for school mental health professionals to conduct with students who are using drugs. However, some emerging approaches—most notably those including MET, CBT, and family-based components (Muck et al., 2001)—are appropriate for adaptation in schools. We have described one such adolescent-focused intervention program and discussed how the model might be adapted for use in a school setting.

A key initial goal in intervening with substance-using students involves working with the students to build motivation and commitment to change their behavior. A number of tools that school mental health professionals can use to help students decide to reduce or stop drug use have been described, with motivational interviewing techniques receiving the most attention. The importance of helping students to develop and practice relapse prevention skills has also been emphasized. CBT techniques and tools have been presented for skill-building intervention sessions as well. Throughout the chapter, we have noted several issues to consider in conducting individual intervention, such as how and when to include family members in the process; the role that school personnel can play when aftercare is being planned or when students are involved in outside treatment; and where to find needed resources. Finally, a case study has illustrated some of the concepts discussed in the chapter. A comprehensive list of resources follows.

CHAPTER RESOURCES

National Clearinghouse for Alcohol and Drug Information
ncadi.samhsa.gov

This government-hosted website offers information through Web links, publications, and educational tip sheets. Here is a samplimg:

- *Keeping Youth Drug-Free: A Guide for Parents, Grandparents, Elders, Mentors, and Other Caregivers* (a free brochure).
- *Student Assistance and the Recovery Process: A Call to Action* and *Helping Addicted Youth Find Recovery* (two webcasts).
- *CSAP Substance Abuse Resource Guide: Middle School and High School Youth.*
- *Tips for Teens* (fact sheets written for youth about drugs and their effects).
- *Let's Help Youth Stay Drug-Free, Part II: Building Healthy Youth: Strategies and Services* (available free as a webcast or by purchase as a videotape or DVD).
- *Suspect Your Teen Is Using Drugs or Drinking?: A Brief Guide to Action for Parents* (booklet with information for parents about talking to their teen about suspected drug use).

Drug Strategies
www.drugstrategies.com

This website offers *Treating Teens: A Guide to Adolescent Drug Programs* (for parents), and a searchable database listing treatment programs nationwide.

Partnership for a Drug-Free America
www.drugfree.org

This site provides information on substances, guides for parents and treatment providers, and resources for teens.

PRIDE Youth Programs
www.prideyouthprograms.org

The organization that runs this site disseminates multimedia materials and curricula for parents, schools, and communities.

Mid-Atlantic Addiction Technology Transfer Center
www.mid-attc.org/adolescent/html/links.htm

This site has a list of electronic resources.

Resources for School-Based Mental Health/Substance Use Treatment

The following centers offer resources, most of which can be downloaded for free from their websites.

- **UCLA School Mental Health Project** (*smhp.psych.ucla.edu*)
- **Center for Adolescent and Family Studies** (*education.indiana.edu/cas/adol/counselor.html*)
- **Center for School Mental Health Analysis and Action** (*csmha.umaryland.edu/resources.html/index.html*)

In addition, the book by Gonet (1994) in the present volume's References list contains excellent information and case examples.

Websites Specifically for Adolescents

- *www.freevibe.com*
- *www.bubblemonkey.com*
- **NIDA for Teens** (*www.teens.drugabuse.gov*)
- *www.thecoolspot.gov*

Select Prevention–Intervention Programs Implemented in School Settings

Materials developed for the following "best-practices" programs may be adaptable for individual interventions implemented by school professionals.

- **Adolescent Transitions Program (ATP)** (*cfc.uoregon.edu/atp.htm*)
- **Strengthening Families Program** (*www.colorado.edu/cspv/blueprints/promising/programs.BPP18.html*)
- **Project Towards No Drug Abuse (TND)** (*tnd.usc.edu*)
- **Reconnecting Youth (RY)** (*www.son.washington.edu/departments/pch/ry*)

Resources for Motivational Interviewing/MET Interventions

Motivational Interviewing
www.motivationalinterview.org

This is the official website of motivational interviewing; it includes general information about links, training resources (including the manual *Motivational Enhancement Therapy with Drug Abusers*), and information on research.

Chestnut Health Systems/Lighthouse Institute
www.chestnut.org/LI/cyt

This site offers clinical materials that were utilized in the CYT study, including the GAIN-Q Full and the PFR.

The following materials in the present book's References list are also helpful: Lambie (2004); Miller and Rollnick (2002); Miller, Zweben, DiClemente, and Rychtarik (1994; this can be obtained through the NCADI website, given above); and Sampl and Kadden (2000; this can also be obtained through the NCADI website).

Resources for CBT Interventions

American Psychiatric Publishing
www.appi.org

Two publications available through this site are recommended for learning more about CBT strategies:

- *Adolescent Substance Abuse Intervention Workbook: Taking a First Step* (by Steven L. Jaffe)
- *Manual of Adolescent Substance Use Treatment* (edited by Todd Wilk Estroff)

The CBT coping skills manual by Kadden et al. (1995) in the present book's References list is also helpful and can be purchased for a nominal fee through the NCADI website.

6

Group Interventions

Group interventions are frequently used in school settings for a number of reasons. First, school mental health professionals can serve a larger number of students in a group format than in individual meetings. Second, for students at the secondary level, their peers gradually become more influential than most adults; thus students can learn from their peers in a group intervention. Third, in groups students learn that peers may be dealing with similar challenges (e.g., substance use, divorce of parents). Finally, groups are more cost-effective than individual meetings with students in terms of school personnel time and resources. Many types of groups can be found in school settings, such as study groups, counseling groups, and advising groups. In this chapter, however, we focus on the types of groups school mental health professionals can facilitate for student substance use and abuse. We review different types of groups, discuss the developmental process of groups, review essential skills needed by group leaders, and highlight the major practical aspects of facilitating groups in schools. As a point of clarification, we use the term *members* throughout this chapter to refer to student members of groups in school settings, and *leader* to refer to the leader of such a group (i.e., a school mental health professional).

TYPES OF GROUP INTERVENTIONS

It is important for school mental health professionals to be aware of the different types of substance-abuse-related groups in which adolescents commonly participate. Some of these groups are appropriate for use in schools, whereas others are more appropriate for use in community settings. The four most common types of groups are psychoeducation, support, self-help, and therapy. Each of these types can be conceptualized along a continuum with "Prevention" at one end and "Treatment" at the other (see Figure 6.1). Psycho-

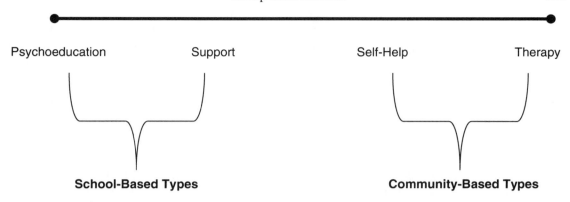

FIGURE 6.1. Continuum of group types for adolescent substance use and abuse.

educational groups fall at the "Prevention" end, whereas therapy groups fall at the "Treatment" end. Support and self-help groups fall somewhere between these two endpoints of the continuum. Each type of group has a different purpose and structure for adolescent members who are dealing with substance-related issues. We now discuss each of these types in more detail.

Psychoeducational Groups

Psychoeducational groups are commonly conducted in schools, where their primary goal is to prevent psychological (e.g., substance abuse, depression) and/or educational (e.g., academic failure) problems. Indeed, in school settings these groups are typically termed *prevention groups*. Most substance abuse prevention programs currently being implemented in U.S. schools incorporate a prevention group component for students. In general, these groups follow a highly structured curriculum and are conducted by a school mental health professional or a teacher specifically trained in the topic area. The group size can range from a few students to an entire class. The format generally consists of providing educational information to the students, as well as including time for discussion and practice of new skills (e.g., drug refusal skills, decision-making skills). These groups are designed to raise student awareness of a problem area such as substance abuse, while imparting practical information about ways to prevent the problem from occurring. They can last for a few weeks, a term, or the entire school year, depending on the length of time needed for the particular group curriculum. It is important to note that these groups are not intended to provide counseling or treatment for an existing substance abuse problem.

Support Groups

As the name implies, the second type of group provides *support* to its members to maintain sobriety or abstinence. In school settings, support groups are typically referred to as *aftercare*; that is, they take place after their members have completed a substance abuse treatment program in the community. Another primary goal of these groups is to help these students succeed in school while refraining from drug use; students returning to a school after attending a substance abuse treatment program typically need support in order to be successful in this setting. Because relapse rates for adolescents completing a substance abuse treatment program are quite high (see Pagliaro & Pagliaro, 1996), providing a support group for these students is an excellent idea. Abstinence from drugs is typically a requirement for support group members; however, students should be able to use the group for support even if relapse occurs.

The leader of a support group is generally a school mental health professional with training in the area of substance abuse, but schools may also contract with a licensed mental health professional (e.g., a social worker) to conduct such a group in the school setting. Support groups are less structured than psychoeducational groups, but leaders can easily implement educational and skill-building components as needed. Group members are encouraged to provide support to each other in such areas as abstaining from drugs, enhancing academic performance, improving interpersonal skills, and dealing with a relapse. In essence, support groups provide recovering student members with a safe place where they can discuss their daily challenges with peers who are experiencing similar problems. It is again important to keep in mind that a support group is *not* considered to be a therapy group. A student should be referred to an outside agency if the school mental health professional believes that a therapy group is warranted (see "Therapy Groups," below). In addition to a school-based support group, students may also be members of self-help groups in the community to support their overall goal of maintaining sobriety or abstinence.

Self-Help Groups

The best-known example of a self-help group for substance abuse is Alcoholics Anonymous (AA). AA groups for both adults and adolescents are commonly found in communities across the nation. Similar groups are available for other drug problems (e.g., Narcotics Anonymous or NA), as well as groups for relatives and friends of persons with a substance abuse problem (including Al-Anon and Alateen). AA and similar groups hold meetings in many locations, such as community centers and church meeting areas. Self-help groups for substance abuse can also be found in hospitals, medical clinics, and community treatment centers.

Typically, the primary goal of self-help groups is to provide support to their members in maintaining sobriety or abstinence. These groups are generally composed of individuals who have experienced or are currently experiencing a particular substance abuse problem. The format of self-help groups can vary from less to more structure, depending on the philosophical model of the group. For example, AA groups are faith-based and rely on a "higher power" in order for members to accomplish the "12 steps" to recovery (see *Chapter 5* for more information on 12-step models). Some self-help groups found in medical settings may be more skill-based in format, in order to provide members with ways to improve how they cope with substance abuse. AA and other 12-step groups are typically facilitated by experienced members who are in recovery from a substance problem, whereas skill-based groups are more likely to be led by mental health professionals. Certain schools or treatment programs will require that adolescents attend a self-help group to support their recovery from substance abuse. As previously suggested, however, self-help groups are most appropriately conducted in the community and *not* the school setting. A common component of substance abuse treatment for adolescents is a therapy group, which we discuss next.

Therapy Groups

Therapy groups are conducted in treatment settings as opposed to schools, but are described here because they are a common component of substance abuse treatment for adolescents (in addition to other treatment modalities, such as individual or family counseling). Treatment programs frequently incorporate the use of groups for adolescents for many of the same reasons they are used in schools. These groups are typically led by a licensed mental health professional (e.g., a social worker, counselor, or psychologist) with expertise in substance abuse treatment. The focus of these groups is on both treating the substance abuse and examining the underlying psychological cause(s) of the problem (e.g., depression, family dysfunction). In general, this type of deeper psychological examination poses more potential risk and reward for its members than do the typical activities of the other group types, and leaders of therapy groups must possess the requisite professional skills and experience to facilitate such groups successfully. In sum, therapy groups are most appropriately conducted as part of a substance abuse treatment program by a licensed mental health professional and *not* in school settings.

As this review has made clear, all groups for student substance use and abuse are not the same, and school mental health professionals should only implement school-based groups that are appropriate for their context and training. More specifically, psychoeducational groups are appropriate for students at risk for substance abuse, whereas support groups are more appropriate for students who have completed substance abuse treatment. In the community, adolescents can access self-help and therapy groups for dealing with substance abuse problems. (It is also important to realize that some students may be members of a school-based support group and a community-based self-help group simultaneously.) School mental health professionals who conduct groups with students on the topic of substance abuse should have an understanding of the developmental process of groups. This is the topic to which we turn next.

UNDERSTANDING THE DEVELOPMENTAL PROCESS OF GROUPS

Groups pass through basic developmental stages during their life spans. We believe that school mental health professionals should have a general understanding of these stages, as it will assist them in better understanding how groups develop and what their leadership role within them should be. The model we present describes four general stages common to the group process, as well as critical issues that should be addressed by the leader and members at each stage (see Figure 6.2). These stages are common to most groups of the four types described above (psychoeducation, support, self-help, therapy); however, they may look different, depending on the purpose of a particular group. For example, discrete stages may be less distinguishable in a highly structured psychoeducation group that meets six times than in a support group that meets for a full school term. In addition, we realize that groups are more dynamic in nature than a stage model suggests, but we also believe that school mental health professionals can use this model as a guide for the developmental process of the groups they facilitate. Readers who have prior experience in facilitating school groups should consider how each of these stages fit with what they have observed. Readers who do not have such experience should think about how they would structure a potential group, based on the following descriptions of stages. Our descriptions here are based on those of Corey and Corey (2006), but are revised for relevancy to secondary school settings.

Initial Stage

The initial stage of a group will take place during the first few meetings, but this stage can begin earlier if the leader conducts a pregroup interview with potential student members (see "Practical Considerations for Group Work in Schools," below, for more on pregroup interviews). Members in the initial stage are new to the group and in the process of deter-

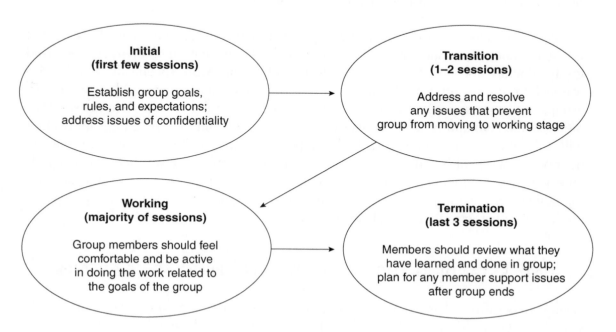

FIGURE 6.2. Stages of group development.

mining what is expected of them, what the purpose of the group is, whether they can trust the leader and other members, how much information they should share, and what they will get out of it. It is thus important for the group leader to provide appropriate amounts of structure during the initial stage, so that members can begin to obtain answers to these questions. In other words, members will be nervous, uncomfortable, and anxious during the initial stage of a group, and the leader should work to make members feel more comfortable by providing reasonable amounts of structure and directly addressing any member concerns. All too often, leaders become frustrated early in the group process because "members are not behaving the way they should." In many instances, poor member participation or presence of negative behaviors (e.g., talking out of turn, criticizing others) is due to the lack of structure and guidance provided by the leader in the initial stage of the group. In addition, negative member behaviors in the initial stage can be due to members' sensing that a leader is not comfortable facilitating the group.

Remember the old adage that "first impressions are important"? Leaders should remember this advice during the initial stage of a group. Adolescent members tend to react more positively to a group leader (and also to the other members) when the leader conveys confidence and enthusiasm for facilitating the group. One of us (Burrow-Sanchez) teaches the group counseling course in his academic department to future school counselors. Typically, during the first class meeting he encounters a few students who indicate their fear of leading groups, especially a group of adolescents! He points out to these students that adolescents can easily detect when a leader is not comfortable facilitating a group. In addition, he advises that having an uncomfortable leader generally gets any group off to a bad start. Thus we recommend that school mental health professionals with little or no experience in leading groups seek out appropriate training and supervision in order to develop their skills and confidence in this area.

During the initial stage of a group, a leader should provide members with a clear statement of the group's purpose—for example, "The purpose of this group is to provide support to fellow students who have just completed substance abuse treatment, so that they can be successful in school and in their lives." The leader should also establish expectations and group rules for member behavior both inside and outside the group. These behavioral expectations should be established early in the initial stage, preferably in the first meeting. Greenberg (2003) provides these examples of group rules: Members maintain confidentiality, begin and end meetings on time, display respectful behavior to other members and the leader, do not talk negatively about others (e.g., peers, teachers) not in the group, agree to attend every group meeting, and do not interrupt others while they are speaking. The leader should clearly convey which rules are non-negotiable, such as those concerning confidentiality and respectful behavior. However, members should be provided with opportunities to discuss each rule and to make suggestions for additional rules relevant for the particular group.

Confidentiality is one of the most important issues to bring up in the initial stage of a group, as part of the discussion of behavioral expectations and group rules. The leader should explain that he or she cannot guarantee confidentiality in a group, because he or she cannot prevent a member from talking about the group to others outside of the group. The leader should then engage members in a discussion on establishing a rule that everyone can agree upon to protect member confidentiality. There can also be a discussion of what the consequences should be when a member violates the confidentiality rule. (We discuss the issue of confidentiality more fully in the "Practical Considerations . . . " section.)

The leader who addresses behavioral expectations and group rules early in the initial stage is establishing a foundation of safety and trust among group members. It is important to note that these expectations and rules will differ somewhat, depending on the type of group being conducted; for example, confidentiality will be less of an issue in a psychoeducational group than in a support group. Leaders should take care to ensure that expectations and rules match the types of groups they are facilitating.

As mentioned above, it is common during the initial stage for members to experience discomfort and anxiety, especially if they have not participated in a group before. Some of this early discomfort can be attributed to the newness of the experience and to the unfamiliarity of at least some other members. A common approach to having members get to know each other better and reduce discomfort during the initial stage is to ask them to engage in an "icebreaker" activity. This activity could include having members pair up, having the members in each pair spend 5 minutes getting acquainted, and then asking each person in a pair to introduce the other person to the group. Many resources provide examples of techniques to use during the initial (and other stages) of a group; we suggest that interested readers consult Corey, Corey, Callanan, and Russell (2004) and Greenberg (2003) for more information. Successfully addressing the important issues described above in the initial stage will allow the group to progress more smoothly to and through the next stage.

Transition Stage

In the transition stage, group members move from understanding the purpose of the group and expectations of them (as presented in the initial stage) to the actual work they are expected to do in the group. Some groups may pass through this stage relatively quickly, whereas others may get stuck here for some time. If the group remains stuck in this stage for too long, it is likely that the leader and members will become frustrated by the lack of progress. When this occurs, members may begin challenging the leader on such issues as his or her ability to lead the group and the importance of the group's purpose. Challenges to the leader are more likely to occur if the group has not adequately addressed the initial-stage issues described above.

Two particular reasons why groups may get stuck in the transition stage are that issues of confidentiality and member expectations may not have been adequately addressed. For example, if members do not clearly understand how confidentiality will be dealt with in the group, there is a high likelihood that trust will be slow to develop, because members may be worried that personal information will be leaked outside the group. In addition, members are less likely to participate fully if they are unclear about the group's purpose and its relation to the problems they are dealing with; adolescents will want to know that a group has personal relevance for their lives. One way to address this issue is to have members develop personal goals for the group in the initial stage (we discuss personal goals more fully in "Practical Considerations . . . "). The bottom line is that if members resist moving past the initial stage, the leader should first assess and then address any potential underlying issues that may be serving as obstacles to the group's development, such as confidentiality or lack of trust. Strategies for dealing with these issues include initiating a straightforward discussion about the leader's observations of member behavior (e.g., lack of participation) that are obstructing group movement. If these issues are dealt with by the leader and members early, the group will spend less time in transition and move more quickly to the working stage.

Working Stage

The working stage is probably what most people think of when they think of group interventions. This is the stage in which the leader and members are actually doing what is needed to achieve the goals of the group. In psychoeducational groups, this may be the stage during which members are practicing newly learned skills (e.g., role playing) in front of other group members. In support groups, this may be the stage in which members are openly providing support and feedback to each other. From the leader's perspective, the working stage is more evident as members become increasingly comfortable with taking a significant role in the educational or skill-based activities of the group, and earlier issues (e.g., confidentiality, trust) are discussed less. (It is important to note that concerns related to confidentiality can emerge at any stage of a group and should be addressed by the leader when they come up.) Members in the working stage also take more ownership of the group, and the leader may find his or her role becoming less prescriptive than in earlier stages; however, this will vary according to the type of group. Toward the end of the working stage, the leader should begin the process of making members aware that the group will end in the near future.

Termination Stage

At least three meetings before a group ends, the leader should begin discussing the process of termination. How a group ends will depend in part on how the group is structured. For example, some groups may be strictly time-limited (e.g., a six-session psychoeducational group), whereas the end of others may coincide with the end of a school term or academic year. Leaders should not assume that all adolescent members know when a group will end, even if a concrete termination date has been established from the beginning.

Raising the issue of termination early is important, because some members may need this prompting in order to participate more fully in the group before its ending. This stage is also a time for members to review what they have learned during the group and what things they will take away from it. Moreover, in a substance abuse support group, the termination stage is a time when members can brainstorm ways to locate and access support after the group ends. Finally, members will have the opportunity to practice relevant behaviors (e.g., drug refusal skills, relapse prevention strategies) and receive feedback before the group ends.

For some groups, there may be the possibility of members' continuing to meet at a predetermined date, such as when a group breaks off at the end of a school term and then begins again the following term. Some schools conduct substance abuse support groups every academic year; therefore, students know they can participate regularly in these groups. The leader may also determine that booster sessions are warranted, in which members meet once or twice after the group ends to check in with and provide support to each other. In addition, the termination stage is a good time for the leader to determine whether any members will need referrals for other services. For example, some students in an aftercare group for substance abuse may require additional support over the summer and may be referred to a self-help group in the community.

A Note about Group Stages

We acknowledge that our discussion of group stages may be perceived as too simplistic. In fact, our own experiences have taught us that groups are more dynamic and fluid than these stages suggest. However, we have provided this discussion as a general framework for understanding the developmental process of groups. We hope that readers of this book do not take the stages above at face value, but rather conceptualize them in terms of their own experiences when conducting groups. In addition to understanding how groups develop over time, leaders should possess specific skills in order to be effective group facilitators.

GROUP LEADERSHIP SKILLS

We firmly believe that a large part of any group's success can be attributed to the skill and confidence of its leader. As noted above, many graduate students in school counseling are initially hesitant about leading groups. Most of these students overcome their initial fear and come to enjoy facilitating groups in schools after receiving training in this area. If you are a school mental health counselor who is new to group work, we suggest that you look for opportunities in your school or district to receive training and supervision in order to develop your skills in this area. Even if you are not new to group work, we suggest you continue to look for ways to improve your skills as a group leader by attending conferences, participating in workshops, or gaining other continuing education experiences. In this section, we discuss the major skills that school mental health professionals need in order to facilitate successful groups in school settings. We realize that our list is not exhaustive, but it includes the skills we believe are critical. Other resources provide additional information on skill development for group leaders (see Corey et al., 2004; Corey & Corey, 2006; Greenberg, 2003).

Basic Counseling Skills

Most graduate students in school-related mental health fields take a course in *basic counseling skills* (BCS) during the first year of their training program. This skill set is also referred to as *intentional interviewing skills* (see Ivey & Ivey, 2003) and *active communication skills* (see Westra, 1996). Regardless of its name, this is a basic set of core competencies for successful interpersonal work. These skills are used in both individual and group counseling, but we focus here on their application to group work. We are keeping our discussions brief, because we assume that much of this material will be familiar to many readers of this chapter; if not, there are many excellent resources on this topic (see Corey & Corey, 2006; Ivey & Ivey, 2003; Westra, 1996).

Active Listening

Among the central components of BCS are *active listening skills* with group members. Active listening skills involve the leader actually hearing and appropriately responding to what members say in the group. This includes hearing not only *what* members say, but *how* they say it. For example, a student in a group may be discussing a past negative event, but his or her body language may not match the content of what is being said. A leader who is actively listening to the student will detect the incongruence between the student's content and body language. The leader can then decide how he or she will comment on this observation. Most students appreciate it when they feel that a leader has actually listened to them and then appropriately responded. Active listening by the leader will encourage members to speak in the group; it also provides an effective model of communication skills for members. For example, the leader can respond to a member by paraphrasing, summarizing, or asking the member for clarification if he or she does not fully understand what has been said (see "Paraphrasing and Summarization," below).

Rapport Building

Rapport building includes all of the subtle things that a leader does to make members feel comfortable in a group. For example, the leader can say such things as "Hi, Tom, I'm glad that you came to the group today," or "Thanks, everyone, for making it to the group on time today." Rapport building also includes the leader's body language, such as facing a student when he or she is speaking or providing appropriate amounts of eye contact. In groups, chairs are typically arranged in a circle, which provides the opportunity for all members and the leader to clearly see each other. Vocal skills are also important and include the way a leader speaks to members (e.g., tone, body posture, facial expression), as well as the clarity of the message.

An important caveat is that the leader must match rapport-building behaviors with the cultural backgrounds of the students in the group. For example, it may be inappropriate for a leader to expect some Hispanic students to make direct eye contact when speaking (see the "Cultural Awareness and Competency" section for the reason). Of course, this statement is itself a cultural assumption and should always be evaluated in regard to the specific cultural characteristics of the students in a group. The main point is that leaders should utilize rapport-building behaviors that are culturally appropriate for group members. We provide sources of information on cultural issues in the "Chapter Resources" section.

Effective Use of Closed- and Open-Ended Questions

Leaders ask questions in order to obtain information from members in a group, and the types of questions leaders ask will determine the types of information they obtain. *Closed-ended questions* are used to obtain specific pieces of information, such as "What grade are you in?" or "What is your second-period class?" Such questions generally can be answered in one or two words. *Open-ended questions* are used by leaders to obtain more meaningful information from members; and they cannot be answered with a couple of words and require the student to respond in more detail. Examples of open-ended questions include "What types of support do you need from members of this group in order to stay away from drugs?" or "What do you mean when you say, 'I can handle problems on my own without this support group'?"

At the beginning of a group, students are typically more comfortable answering closed-ended questions than open-ended questions. As the group progresses, however, members will gradually become more comfortable responding to open-ended questions. Some students will require more practice in responding to open-ended questions than others. The leader should consider this last statement in regard to the developmental level of the group members; older students (i.e., high school) are likely to have more cognitive capacity for responding to both types of questions than younger students (i.e., middle school). Furthermore, students with poor communication skills will initially experience frustration and difficulty in responding to open-ended questions. At the beginning of a group, the leader should casually assess the communication skills of each group member, in order to determine which types of questions will produce the least amount of discomfort during the initial meetings. This information can also be used by the leader to determine which communication skills specific members should work on as the group progresses.

Paraphrasing and Summarization

As noted above in connection with active listening, *paraphrasing* and *summarization* are two important skills for a leader to master, because they communicate to group members that the leader has truly listened to what has been said. Paraphrasing involves the leader briefly repeating back the message of what a member has said by integrating the member's own words with the leader's words (Ivey & Ivey, 2003). Summarization is similar to paraphrasing but involves the leader including more information, typically from more than one person in the group, in order to clarify and organize what has been said (Ivey & Ivey, 2003). By using both of these skills, a leader not only allows members to feel heard in the group, but also has the opportunity to ask for clarification of the message. Consider the following example of a leader's use of paraphrasing with a student in a group:

PARKER (STUDENT MEMBER): Things have been really tough lately, and everyone is on my back! Ever since I got busted for having marijuana, people have been on my case! My parents just don't understand and think I'm some pothead, and they don't listen to me when I tell them I'm not. I think my teachers know that I was busted for pot, because they have been treating me differently, like I'm some type of troublemaker. Things really suck, and I wish people would just treat me like other kids, because I'm not the only one in this school who smokes pot. I was just the one who got caught!

LEADER: Parker, sounds like you are saying that things are tough for you right now, especially because you feel as if your parents and teachers are treating you differently due to your recently being caught with marijuana. Does that sound about right to you?

PARKER: Yeah, totally! See, you get it! Why can't other people?

In this example, the leader briefly paraphrases the content of Parker's message and then includes a tag question ("Does that sound about right to you?") to make sure that he or she has heard the message correctly. Including a tag question at the end of a paraphrase is a good way for a leader to indicate the importance to understand the content of what a member has said. Such a question also provides the member with the opportunity to affirm the leader's paraphrased statement or amend it.

In contrast to paraphrasing, summarization can be used by a leader to clarify and organize what many members have said, as well as to make a transition into another topic. In the next example, all members of a substance abuse support group have just finished briefly checking in at the beginning of the group session and providing a brief overview of their week since the previous group meeting. Consider how the leader of this group uses summarization:

"I want to thank everyone for checking in and letting us know how your week has gone since our last group meeting. Sounds like there are a lot of similarities in what each of you have said. Quite a few of you mentioned feeling overworked with school assignments as the term is coming to an end. I also heard many of you say that you are working hard to deal with the stress of your workload in ways that are healthier than using drugs, which is what many of you have done in the past. Based on what you all have said, I think it may be a good idea if we spend some time during the group today to discuss what members have been doing to successfully manage their stress and how the group can support them in staying clean from drugs. How does that sound to everyone?"

In this example, the leader summarizes the content of what members have said during the check-in period. The leader then uses this summarization as a springboard for a transition into a relevant topic for that particular group meeting. She also includes a tag question to allow members to respond to the summarization before moving on. Although we have provided some examples of how to use the skills of paraphrasing and summarization, readers will discover many useful variations of these skills as they facilitate groups. For more information, readers are encouraged to consult the references on BCS cited at the beginning of this section.

Modeling Desired Behaviors

As discussed in Chapter 2, one of the most powerful methods of learning is watching others model or perform a behavior. Most substance-abuse-related groups will include some teaching of appropriate behaviors or skills to the student members, such as decision making, problem solving, social skills, or a combination of all these. Leaders will need to be able to provide good models of the behaviors or skills to be taught, and thus they should be well practiced in these. At the beginning of a group, members will look to the leader for guidance and will also be observing how he or she interacts with group members. The behavior of the leader at the beginning of a group will set the stage for how the group progresses. For example, the leader can make members either feel heard in the group through the appropriate use of paraphrasing and summarization, or feel disrespected by responding sarcastically to what they say.

Because the influence of the leader's behavior will be stronger at the beginning of the group, it is important for leaders to show congruence between what they say and how they act from the beginning. For example, if a leader says that disrespectful behavior by members will not be tolerated in the group, he or she should not engage in this behavior either. As the group progresses, members will become more comfortable in pointing out discrepancies between the leader's words and actions, as well as those of other members. In sum, it is important for leaders to be good models for behavior they expect group members to display.

Confrontation

The word *confrontation* typically conjures up images of people yelling at each other about an issue on which they do not agree. Although such images may be a bit dramatic, confrontation is not usually associated with something positive. Most people, even school mental health professionals, typically like to avoid confronting others because it makes them feel uncomfortable. However, we encourage our readers to reconceptualize confrontational behavior in a more positive and constructive manner, because they will use it in groups. Group leaders will need to hone their skills at confronting members—but the way in which they do this will make the difference between inviting an argument or encouraging a member to examine his or her own behavior thoughtfully.

We define *confrontation* as a leader's (or another member's) pointing out a discrepancy between what a member says and what he or she does. For example, in a school-based substance abuse support group for students, a student named Amanda says, "I know that staying clean is important, but every time I go to a party I end up smoking some pot with my friends. I guess that's just the way it is for me." She then goes on to discuss another topic. The leader of this group, can either ignore Amanda's comment or use a confrontation strategy to address it with her. A confrontation strategy may sound something like this: "Hold on a minute, Amanda. You just said that staying clean is important to you, but then you went on to stay that you smoke pot at parties. So I'm a bit confused about how important it is for you to stay clean if you are continuing to smoke pot. Can you explain that a bit more for me?" As you can see, the leader points out the discrepancy in Amanda's statement, expresses confusion, and then asks her to elaborate. This type of confrontation has the benefit of allowing Amanda to become aware of the discrepancy between her goals (remaining clean) and actions (smoking pot at parties) in relation to substance abuse. In addition, the confrontation strategy indicates to Amanda that the leader is actively listening to what she says by stopping her and pointing out the discrepancy, rather than just letting her go on to some other topic. Leaders who use confrontation in a constructive manner such as this will not only serve as good models for communication skills, but will also assist members in increasing their awareness of the discrepancies between goals and behaviors.

Working with Resistant Members

It goes without saying that some adolescent members of a substance-abuse-related group will not want to be in the group. Those of us in the mental health professions like to believe that members come to our groups motivated and willing to participate; however, this is not always the case, especially when working with adolescents. Leaders, should anticipate that some members will display behaviors that indicate their resistance to being in a group. Both voluntary and involuntary group members can exhibit resistant behaviors (see the later section "Attendance" for more information on involuntary members). These types of behaviors include remaining silent, providing limited responses to questions, verbally indicating that they do not need to be in the group, and constantly challenging the leader or other members.

Experience has taught us that group leaders will be better equipped to deal with resistant member behaviors if they both anticipate resistance and have some general ideas about how to address it. Among the most useful techniques we have found for working with resistant adolescents are those of *motivational interviewing* (Miller & Rollnick, 1991, 2002). Although many leaders do not feel comfortable dealing directly with resistant member behavior when it occurs in a group, the developers of motivational interviewing suggest that a leader should address member resistance directly rather than avoiding it. The leader should view resistant behavior as a signal that something is going on with a member that needs to be addressed in the group. It is important for the leader to determine what is causing the resistance rather than immediately providing negative consequences (e.g., removal from the group). Dealing with resistant member behaviors in an appropriate manner will not only prevent further disruption and member dropout, but will enhance the quality of the working relationships within a group.

It is true that resistant behaviors are some of the most challenging leaders will encounter in groups of adolescents. However, it is very important not to become defensive in the face of resistant behaviors. This is sometimes difficult for adults to do when working with adolescents, because they may feel as if "I am in charge" and "I know better than the students." Nevertheless, a leader who works on understanding why a student is engaging in resistant behavior rather than punishing it will be more likely to address it constructively without letting defensiveness get in the way. Useful questions include "Why is the member acting like this?" and "What is his or her resistant behavior telling me?" The leader can then use many of the communication skills described above to deal with the behavior. To make these concepts clearer, let's take a look at how one group leader addresses resistant behavior:

> TREVON (STUDENT MEMBER): I hate being in this stupid group! I think it's a waste of time, because we don't do anything! I'm tired of listening to other people's problems when they don't have anything to do with me!
>
> LEADER: Trevon, it sounds like that you don't like being in the group because you feel it is a waste of your time, and some of the things we talk about don't have anything to do with you. Am I hearing you correctly?
>
> TREVON: Yeah, that's about right.
>
> LEADER: I understand what you're saying. I agree, I wouldn't want to be in a group that I didn't feel was benefiting me and was a waste of my time. I'm sorry that you feel this way, but I am also glad that you are letting us know how you feel about being in the group. You know that we want the group to have some benefit for everyone in it. So can you help us understand ways the group can be more beneficial to you?

In this example, the leader addresses Trevon's resistant behavior through the use of paraphrasing and summarization, and also gives him the opportunity to explore the reasons why he feels dissatisfied about being in the group. Alternatively, the leader could easily respond by saying, "Trevon, I don't like your attitude and think what you said is disrespectful. Why don't you sit out this group and think about it?" or "Okay, Trevon, since you don't want to be in the group and it's a waste of time for you, then please leave! We don't want to waste your time!" These types of responses would not provide the opportunity to engage Trevon further, but instead would shut down the communication process. More information about effective ways to manage resistant behavior from the perspective of motivational interviewing are available in the "Chapter Resources" section, as well as in the book's list of references.

Cultural Awareness and Competency

Students in U.S. schools come from many different cultural backgrounds. We believe that as schools become more diverse, school mental health professionals have the opportunity to broaden their cultural worldviews and further develop skill sets that take students' cultural backgrounds into account. We acknowledge that training in topics related to student diversity or multicultural competency is a relatively new phenomenon in graduate programs, and thus many school mental health professionals may not have received this training during their formal education. In some instances, schools or districts have provided school mental health professionals with training in this area, and we applaud them for doing so. We also want to stress that training in diversity-related issues is not a one-time event, but should be an ongoing learning experience for all school professionals who work with diverse populations. Although we cannot provide a full discussion of multicultural competency and work with culturally diverse students within the limits of this chapter, we provide a general framework as well as recommendations for additional resources on this topic.

Because group leaders are increasingly likely to have students from different cultural backgrounds in the groups they facilitate, it is important for leaders to be aware of their own attitudes, beliefs, and biases about their own and other cultures. For example, a leader who identifies him- or herself as coming from European American culture is *likely* to espouse such values as individualism, strong work ethic, success measured by job title and money, strong adherence to time-related rules, and the importance of competition. We realize that this sentence includes some oversimplifications of European American culture, but we are trying to make the point that each culture has its own unique set of values, beliefs, and biases, some of which may differ from those of other cultures. Leaders who are aware of their own cultural values, beliefs, and biases will be able to work more effectively with students whose cultural backgrounds are different from their own.

Leaders should also be aware of the ways in which the cultural values and beliefs of students in their groups may differ from their own. For example, families from various Hispanic backgrounds may share the belief that success of interpersonal relationships among family members are more important than the success of an individual person. Such a belief reflects a collectivistic perspective, as opposed to an individualistic perspective (which is typical of European American culture). This type of cultural awareness about others is important for group leaders to develop in order to effectively facilitate groups of culturally diverse students.

Although we believe that developing multicultural competency is a lifelong process, school mental health professionals can do several things to improve their skills in this area. To address this issue, we offer the following three guidelines. We realize that our readers will all be at slightly different places in terms of multicultural competency; therefore, we encourage each of you to consider how these three guidelines relate to your own current level of such competency. We have based the guidelines on the work of Sue and colleagues (1998).

1. *Know yourself.* It is important for you as a group leader to have a good sense of yourself as a cultural being. That is, all of us identify with a specific culture (or cultures), which espouses particular values, beliefs, and biases and influences us in many ways. The more you understand about your own culture(s), the more aware you will be of the values, beliefs, and biases that guide your thinking and behavior.

2. *Know the student populations you work with.* It is unrealistic to expect that school mental health professionals will know everything about every cultural group. However, it is important for such professionals to be aware of the values, beliefs, and practices of culturally different students in their schools. For example, your school may have a large Hispanic student population. If this is true, and if you are not Hispanic, then we suggest you make a commitment to yourself to learn about the Hispanic culture(s) specific to the students at your school (Puerto Rican, Mexican, Cuban, etc.). This can include reading relevant resources on the topic, attending functions in the local Hispanic community, or finding a cultural mentor. A *cultural mentor* is another adult who is familiar with the particular culture you want to learn more about and can help you in this process. It is ideal if you can find a cultural mentor who is also a school mental health professional, since he or she will be familiar with the issues you are dealing with in a school setting.

3. *Know the most culturally relevant skills, interventions, and techniques.* Most substance abuse prevention and intervention programs for students are based on the values and beliefs of the dominant European American culture. This means that many of these interventions are based on the values, beliefs, and practices of this culture and may not be appropriate for use with students from culturally different groups. For example, many substance abuse prevention and intervention programs include components for enhancing students' communication skills. As part of developing these skills, students are commonly taught ways to improve communication with their parents. Frequently, one thing they are taught is to make direct eye contact when speaking with others. Learning this skill may work well for students from the dominant culture, because it is considered respectful in this culture to "look someone in the eyes" when speaking to him or her. This same skill may not be appropriate, and may possibly even damage a parent–child relationship, for a student from a culturally different background. The parents of a Hispanic student, for example, may consider the use of direct eye contact by their son or daughter to be very disrespectful; this could worsen, not improve, communication between the student and his or her parents. Thus leaders who are not aware of the values, beliefs, and practices of culturally different students may inadvertently use interventions or teach skills that are not appropriate for some of these students. In sum, we suggest that the programs and learning materials used in groups should take into account cultural variations among students. If culturally sensitive materials are not readily available, then the standard group curriculum may need to be adapted in various ways. More information on culturally sensitive group curricula and other cultural issues is available in the "Chapter Resources" section.

As discussed above, your skills as a leader are very important for the effective facilitation of groups. We suggest that you take an inventory of the skills described above and assess how competent you feel in each area. Then make a list of the areas in which you could further develop your skills and prioritize them. After making this list, we urge you to make a commitment to develop your skills further in each area, beginning with the highest priority and working down the list as time and resources permit. One way to begin this process is to consult with a more experienced group leader about ways you can develop your skills in the areas identified on your list. We know that the investment you make in improving your leadership skills will greatly benefit the future groups you conduct. In addition to the specific skills discussed above, various practical issues need to be considered in planning to conduct a group.

PRACTICAL CONSIDERATIONS OF GROUP WORK IN SCHOOLS

Conducting groups in a school setting provides its own set of practical challenges for school mental health professionals. These challenges include everything from finding adequate space for group sessions to ensuring that members attend them. In this section, we discuss the many practical considerations involved in conducting groups in schools. Our readers may already be aware of some of these issues and not others; however, we believe that they are all important to consider. As you read this section, think about how these considerations apply to your specific situation and ways you would successfully negotiate them.

Developing a Group Plan

It is important for a school mental health professional to have a structured plan for conducting a group with adolescent students. Such a plan not only provides a "roadmap" for the leader, but allows him or her to consider the structure of the group before it begins. One of the most common mistakes that new leaders make is to assume that they can "get by" facilitating a group of adolescents with little thought about its structure. These leaders quickly find that providing little structure for members makes the task of facilitating a group much harder. In fact, having a plan for the group is likely to help a leader as much as it does the student members. At a minimum, group plans should be outlines that indicate the topics and activities to be covered during each group meeting. Highly developed group plans are detailed manuals that leaders follow, and possibly corresponding workbooks for the members. The level of detail needed for a group plan will depend on the type of group, the leader's skill and comfort levels, and the content to be covered during the group. In general, persons new to leading groups will prefer more detailed plans, whereas more experienced individuals will be more comfortable with less detailed plans.

Several manuals have been developed for addressing adolescent substance abuse issues in group and individual settings; we have also found that many of the individually based manuals can easily be adapted to group formats (see the "Chapter Resources" section for information on group curricula). Therefore, leaders can probably find a manual to draw upon in constructing a group plan for use in a school setting. They may find, however, that some group manuals do not exactly fit with their own school settings. In these cases, they may want to adapt a previously developed group manual for their settings or develop their own group plan based on a compilation of manuals. To address this latter issue, we provide five steps below for use in developing or adapting a group plan. We have based our own sample outline (see Figure 6.3) on the development of a substance abuse support group for high school students, but similar guidelines can be used for a psychoeducational group.

1. *Determine purpose and goals for the group.* In our Figure 6.3 example, the *purpose* of the group is to support high school students in maintaining abstinence and improve academic success in the school setting. It is assumed that students in this group will have completed a substance abuse treatment program in the community. The *goals* of the group are to (1) assist members in recognizing signs of relapse; (2) improve problem-solving, decision-making, and communication skills to negotiate stressors that threaten abstinence; and (3) improve academic skills (e.g., studying, test taking) so that school becomes more rewarding.

2. *Determine group logistics.* As outlined in Figure 6.3, the group leader will conduct a pregroup interview with potential group members and their parents, in order to explain the purpose of the group and to address issues of student/parental consent. The group will be time-limited to 10 sessions (with an option of extending to 12, if needed) and will start at the beginning of the school term with a total of six to eight students. The group will meet on a weekly basis for a regular class period in Room 334 (the group leader has confirmed that Room 334 is available for the group during the term). The group will meet on a rotating class period schedule throughout the term; that is, the first meeting will take place during first period, the second meeting the following week during second period, and so forth (the meeting cycle will begin anew after the last class period is reached).

3. *Determine content for each meeting.* The specific content for each group meeting is based on the purpose and goals identified above, and is indicated in the group outline (see Figure 6.3). The content will be adapted from preexisting research-based manuals on adolescent substance abuse.

4. *Determine learning activities for each meeting.* The learning activities are directly based on the content to be covered in each meeting (again, see Figure 6.3). They are designed to teach members the related skills of each content area. Learning activities will be adapted from preexisting research-based manuals on adolescent substance abuse.

5. *Determine way(s) to evaluate group outcomes.* Based on the purpose and goals of the group, outcomes will be evaluated in the following ways: (1) members' reports of substance use–nonuse as rated on a 14-item measure of alcohol and drug use, administered before the group begins and after it ends (Moberg, 2000); (2) members' reports of coping with stressful substance-abuse-related situations as rated on a 33-item coping measure, administered before the group begins and after it ends (Myers, Brown, & Mott, 1993); (3) comparison of grade point average (GPA) and school attendance for each member from the term prior to group participation to the term of group participation, and a one-term

Group Purpose: Support group to help students with substance abuse maintain abstinence and increase academic success. (Assumption: Students will have completed a substance abuse treatment program in the community.)

Group Goals: (1) Assist members in recognizing and managing signs of relapse; (2) improve problem-solving, decision-making, and communication skills, to help members negotiate stressors that threaten abstinence; and (3) improve academic skills (e.g., studying, test taking) so that school becomes more rewarding.

Group Logistics: At least 10 sessions (with option of extending to 12 if needed), with a total of six to eight student members. Pregroup interview to be conducted with each student and parent(s). Group to meet on a weekly basis for a regular class period, with a rotating class period schedule throughout the duration of the group.

Outline of Group Content and Learning Activities:

(*Note*: Each session will begin and end with a brief member check-in and check-out, respectively. Homework will be assigned at the end of each meeting to reinforce learning between group meetings.)

1. First Group Meeting
   a. Explain purpose of group.
   b. Provide overview of entire group (10–12 meetings).
   c. Conduct an icebreaker activity.
   d. Discuss issues of confidentiality.

2. Preventing a Relapse
   a. Discuss the triggers (warning signs) to relapse.
   b. Discuss ways to manage triggers.
   c. Role-play substance refusal skills.

3. Managing a Relapse
   a. Review ways to prevent a relapse.
   b. Discuss ways to manage a relapse, if it occurs.
   c. Discuss importance of seeking support after a relapse.
   d. Each member develops a plan for coping with a relapse.

4. Improving Problem-Solving/Decision-Making Skills (Part 1)
   a. Discuss substance-related problems members face.
   b. Discuss both good and bad examples of solving problems.
   c. Teach brainstorming strategy for successfully solving problems.
   d. Present various problem-solving scenarios to members, and have them implement brainstorming strategy to solve each one.

(continued)

FIGURE 6.3. Outline for a student aftercare group.

5. Improving Problem-Solving/Decision-Making Skills (Part 2)
   a. Review material from last group meeting.
   b. Continue presenting various problem-solving scenarios to members, and have them implement brainstorming strategy to solve each one.

6. Improving Communication Skills (Part 1)
   a. Discuss communication problems that members experience.
   b. Discuss both good and bad examples of solving communication problems.
   c. Teach two or three important communication skills relevant to group members.
   d. Ask members to role-play communication skill scenarios.

7. Improving Communication Skills (Part 2)
   a. Review material from previous sessions.
   b. Teach additional one or two communication skills.
   c. Ask members to role-play communication skill scenarios.
   d. Briefly mention that three meetings remain, and ask members to think about what it means to them that the group will end.

8. Improving Academic Skills
   a. Discuss academic challenges members face.
   b. Discuss both good and bad examples of dealing with academic challenges.
   c. Brainstorm what skills from prior meetings can be used to deal appropriately with academic challenges.
   d. Ask members to role-play academic skills scenarios to reinforce learning.
   e. Mention that two meetings remain, and ask for member thoughts about termination.

9. Putting It All Together
   a. Review material and skills covered in previous sessions.
   b. Provide scenarios that members can respond to in order to display the skills they have learned.
   c. Discuss ways members will be able to receive the support they need after group ends.

10. Termination Meeting
   a. Have each member review what he or she has learned from this group.
   b. Have members discuss what substance-use-related challenges they anticipate facing after group ends.
   c. Have each member discuss ways to cope with these challenges after group ends.
   d. Have members discuss what sources of support are available to them both at school and in the community.
   e. If applicable, provide members with information on other relevant groups that will be offered in their school.

11. Optional meeting, if needed.

12. Optional meeting, if needed.

FIGURE 6.3. (*page 2 of 2*)

follow-up period; and (4) members' satisfaction with the group as rated on an 8-item satisfaction measure, administered at the end of the group (Attkisson & Greenfield, 1999).

Group Logistics

As the second of the five steps above indicates, many important logistical issues need to be considered by school mental health professionals before beginning a group. These issues include group size, time, space, pregroup interviews, co-leadership, and attendance. We address each of these in more detail below.

Group Size

There are a number of factors to consider when determining the size of a group. Typically, new group leaders will be more comfortable with smaller groups until they gain experience and expertise. Size will also depend on the space available for the group, as well as the type of group to be conducted. For example, a psychoeducational group on substance abuse prevention can generally be much larger than a support group for students recovering from substance abuse. School counselors frequently do classroom guidance, which could involve leading a psychoeducational substance abuse prevention group with an entire class of students. For substance abuse support groups, we suggest a group size of about six to eight students.

Time and Scheduling

Time and scheduling are always major issues in schools, because there is never enough time to schedule everything that could potentially benefit a student in a typical school day. A group leader will probably need to negotiate with students' teachers about ways to minimize disruption to the students' academic schedule so that they can attend the group. In addition, some teachers may see limited value in students' attending the group compared to attending class. If this is the case, the leader should work on garnering the teachers' support for the students' attending the group (see also "Support from the Larger System," below).

Group meetings at the secondary level are generally scheduled for an entire class period in most schools. One of the common ways to schedule groups is to use a weekly rotating class period schedule, as described in the second step given above. This type of scheduling may be more acceptable to teachers, as it distributes missed classes more evenly throughout the term for students. Of course, we suggest using a scheduling strategy that works best for everyone involved (students, teachers, and the group), and devising such a strategy will usually require much patience and flexibility.

Another important consideration in scheduling a group is to consider the fact that many of the students who will be attending the group may have fallen behind their peers academically. As discussed in Chapter 2, poor academic performance is a risk factor for substance abuse. Missing academic instruction to attend a group may put a student even further behind, which may place him or her at risk for substance abuse. Therefore, one issue that will need to be addressed up front is how students will make up missed classes and assignments when attending the group.

Space

Another major issue in schools is space, because there is never enough of it! Some school counseling departments have a room assigned for groups, but many others do not. If possible, we suggest finding a space in the school that can be used for every group meeting; it is difficult to move a group to different locations in a school building for each meeting. It is also important to find a space that is reasonably quiet and provides privacy for the group, especially if it is a support group. Rooms where outside distractions are kept to a minimum and windows have working blinds are ideal. Finally, the room should be made as inviting and comfortable as possible for students in the group. This can include having a room large enough for chairs to be placed in a circle, providing reasonably comfortable chairs, and removing potentially distracting objects from the room. Doing little things to make the environment more comfortable for members will greatly increase the group's chances of success.

Pregroup Interviews

Conducting pregroup interviews with potential members is an important first step in facilitating an effective group. In a school setting, a pregroup interview should include the student and his or her parent(s). We realize that school mental health professionals typically do not have a lot of extra time to spare, and pregroup interviews often get overlooked; if time permits such interviews, however, we are sure that they will be well worth the initial investment.

The pregroup interview should include explaining the purpose of the group to the student and parent(s), as well as addressing issues of student and parent consent. This interview also provides the opportunity to determine whether the group will be a good fit for a particular student or whether something else seems more appropriate (e.g., referral to a community agency). For example, a student being interviewed for a substance abuse support group may really benefit more from an outpatient treatment group in the community. Finally, the leader can take some time in the pregroup interview to explain the basic structure, rules, and expectations of group membership. Providing this type of information will inform the student and parent(s), as well as prepare the student for what to expect at the first group meeting.

If there is no time to conduct individual pregroup interviews, an alternative is to use the first group meeting as a pregroup interview. That is, the first group meeting serves the same purpose as a pregroup interview, but only includes potential student members. In this case, however, the leader must also either schedule time to meet with each student's parents, or schedule a group meeting for parents in which to explain the group and address consent issues. As a school mental health professional, you should be aware of your school's policies and protocol for obtaining student and parental consent; as a group facilitator, it is important for you to make personal contact with each student's parents, as they can become allies in supporting the purpose and goals of the group.

Co-Leadership

Throughout this chapter, we have discussed facilitating a group from the perspective of a single leader rather than that of co-leadership. In many school settings, another school mental health professional is simply not available to assist in leading a group. If it is feasible, however, a leader may want to consider co-leading a group with a colleague. There are both benefits and drawbacks to co-leading a group, and the decision will depend on what is appropriate for a particular situation. One benefit of co-leadership is simply having another professional present to share in the work of facilitating the group. A co-leader can also provide another perspective for facilitating the group and assist in determining whether the group is progressing toward its goals. For a less experienced group leader, working with an experienced co-leader can be an excellent way to learn and to improve leadership skills. Two possible drawbacks to working with a co-leader include not agreeing on how to facilitate the group and not having complementary interpersonal styles.

If two professionals do decide on using a co-leadership format, then it is a good idea to meet briefly before and possibly after each group meeting, so that they can engage in regular discussion about the group. Obviously, these types of additional meetings take time and can feel burdensome with an already busy schedule, but they also help the leaders stay "on the same page" in co-leading the group. We believe that most of the potential drawbacks of co-leadership can successfully be worked out if both leaders are committed to facilitating a successful group. In other words, we believe that the benefits of co-leadership will usually outweigh any potential drawbacks.

Attendance

School mental health professionals are likely to find that erratic attendance can be an obstacle to members' success in groups. Specifically, students may be absent on the day of a group session or may have teachers who are reluctant to release them from class to attend the group. We suggest that regular attendance should be a requirement for group participation, and that this requirement should be made explicit to students, parents, teachers, and administrators. The goal of this requirement is to assist all parties in seeing that the group is valuable and that nothing can be achieved unless students actually attend the group. The leader of a support group for students dealing with substance abuse can provide parents and teachers with information about the reasons why group participation is important for successful aftercare support. Many parents and teachers are unaware of the high relapse rates and may feel that once a student has been through treatment, follow-up work is unnecessary or unimportant.

Another attendance-related issue is that of voluntary versus involuntary (mandated) attendance. That is, some students may attend the group by choice, whereas others may be required to attend by some authority (e.g., the school administration). Groups can be successful regardless of whether membership is voluntary or involuntary, although students who are mandated to attend a group may initially express more resistance to the group than voluntary members. A leader can potentially address some of these issues as part of the pregroup interview and during the initial group meetings (see also "Working with Resistant Members," above). If enough students are required to attend a group, then perhaps there can be one group composed of mandated students and another of voluntary students. It is important to consider how to address the issues of involuntary attendance with group members, as these are likely to come up at the beginning of the group.

Confidentiality

Confidentiality is yet another important issue to consider in conducting groups. As suggested earlier in the chapter, leaders should address the issue of confidentiality in the initial group meetings and as required thereafter. In particular, students in a substance abuse support group will be less likely to share information if they do not know what will happen to that information. Common questions include "Will the leader tell my parents about what I say in the group?", "Will I get in more trouble by talking about my drug use?", and "Will other students in the group talk with their friends about what I say in here?" These are all important questions that must be addressed by the group leader, even if the group members do not feel comfortable asking them openly at the beginning of the group. Appropriately addressing confidentiality early in the group will provide a foundation for trust among members and between the leader and members. We provide the following guidelines to assist school mental health professionals in addressing issues of confidentiality in groups.

Understanding School Policies and Laws

Group leaders should clearly understand their schools' policies and appropriate laws (at both state and federal levels) for dealing with issues of confidentiality related to substance abuse (see Chapter 1 for more information). If a group leader has any questions about applicable policies and laws, he or she should consult with another professional who is knowledgeable in this area prior to beginning a group.

Contacting Students and Parents before the Group Begins

At some point before the group begins (the best time is during a pregroup interview if such an interview is possible), the group leader should make personal contact with each student and his or her parent(s) to explain the purpose of the group, obtain consent, and discuss issues of confidentiality. Ideally, the parent(s) and student will both be present at this meeting, so that they can hear the same message regarding confidentiality. The leader will need to communicate to the student and parent(s) what will and will not be shared outside of the group and with whom, depending on the school's policies and applicable laws. Consider the following example during a pregroup interview:

> MOTHER OF STUDENT: So will you tell us if Jake [her son] is using drugs? I bet he will talk about this in the group, and I think it's important that we know what's going on.

> LEADER: I can understand why you think it is important to know about Jake's drug use. You seem to care for him a great deal, and since he has just returned to school after completing a substance abuse treatment program, I know that you want to make sure he stays on the right track.

> MOTHER: Yeah, I want him to stop using drugs. It has caused our family a lot of trouble.

> LEADER: Well, as I have already explained, the purpose of this group is to provide support to students who are trying to stay clean after completing a substance abuse treatment program. Also, as I've mentioned, there are certain times when I have to report information outside of the group—such as when I hear information that leads me to believe Jake is at risk for hurting himself or someone else, or in cases of suspected child abuse. However, I also know from working with adolescents in support groups that they will benefit more when they feel comfortable sharing information that they know will not go outside of the group. This type of information typically includes past or present drug use, as well as the challenges they experience in staying clean. One of the goals of the group is to provide student members with a safe place to express what they are experiencing related to dealing with substances and help them overcome obstacles to their abstinence. With that in mind, we have talked about how I typically only share attendance information with parents of students in the group. That is, I will let you know each week whether or not Jake has attended the group. How does that sound to you?

> MOTHER: Well, I guess that sounds okay. I can understand why you set it up that way.

> LEADER: If there's ever a point in which you don't feel comfortable with that arrangement, then we can all meet again and discuss it further. How does that sound?

> MOTHER: Okay, that sounds better.

This example illustrates how the group leader discusses the issue of confidentiality with Jake's mother—specifically, the question of what type of information will and will not be shared outside the group. Since this is a pregroup interview, Jake is present and hears the same information, which places everyone "on the same page" regarding confidentiality. The leader also leaves the door open to discuss this issue, if needed, in the future. Of course, the leader has made this arrangement with the parent and student within the context of applicable policies and laws concerning confidentiality in this particular school setting.

Discussing Confidentiality at the First Group Meeting

As we have stressed throughout this chapter, the issue of confidentiality should be discussed with members at the first group meeting and as needed thereafter. The leader should be explicit in this discussion, with a particular focus on what types of information will and will not be shared outside the group. Also, the leader should inform members that he or she cannot guarantee confidentiality in a group setting. That is, he or she cannot control whether a member talks with others about things that happen in the group. Given this, we strongly suggest that the leader implement a rule about confidentiality, along with the other group rules. The leader should provide members with explicit examples of what types of information can and cannot be shared with others outside the group, based on the confidentiality rule. The leader may also want to have a discussion with the group about what type of consequences will be imposed if a member violates the confidentiality rule. Talking openly and explicitly about issues of confidentiality will go a long way to create trust and promote free discussion in any group.

Member Goals

We think it is good practice to have members develop goals for themselves related to the purpose of the group—ideally, during the first or second group meeting. Goal setting encourages members to consider thoughtfully what they want to get out of the group. This may be especially important for involuntary members, who may initially think that attending the group is a punishment imposed by adults in authority rather than a valuable activity. For example, after covering the purpose of the group in the initial meeting, the leader can ask members to think about what they would like to get from the group, and then to develop two or three goals prior to the next meeting. The leader should provide explicit examples of appropriate and inappropriate goals, as some members will struggle with this assignment. Some members may express such goals as "I want to stay off drugs," whereas others may say things like "I just want to get out of class." If students express goals similar to the latter, we suggest teaching them how to make their goals more meaningful. The leader can also engage the group members in this process by having them model appropriate and inappropriate goal setting.

Setting goals can be helpful not only in the group's initial stage, but in tracking members' progress throughout the group. Consider the following example:

LEADER (SESSION 5): Leslie, at the beginning of the group, you said that one of your goals was to learn ways to stay away from drugs. How has that been going for you? Has your participation in the group been helping you with that?

LESLIE: I've been having some problems with that. I mean that I am not as clean as I wanted to be when I made that goal. So I guess that my goal hasn't been working so good, but I still want to work on it.

LEADER: Leslie, thanks for letting us know how things have been going for you related to your goal. Sounds like you've been struggling a bit with your goal, but it is still important to you. Can you tell us in what ways the group can help you in achieving your goal?

LESLIE: I guess one thing would be if people could ask me more often about how my goal is going. That way, it would remind me to stay on top of it more.

In this example, the leader reminds Leslie of one of her goals, and also checks in on her progress toward achieving it. Finding that Leslie has been struggling with this particular goal, the leader is able to begin a discussion on ways the group can support her in working toward it. If Leslie was not able to generate ideas for support from the group, then the leader could call upon other members for input.

Support from the Larger System

In order for school mental health professionals to maintain the ability to facilitate groups over time, support from stakeholders (e.g., administrators, teachers, parents) in the larger system is needed. We suggest finding ways to demonstrate to these stakeholders that the groups you facilitate are a valuable asset for students. Group leaders can do this by making personal connections with other school personnel and explaining the rationale and importance of providing groups for students. We have also emphasized above the importance of establishing personal contact with the parents of group members. In addition, we have provided ideas for obtaining outcome data for groups (see "Developing a Group Plan," above). Presenting meaningful outcome data to colleagues and administrators will go a long way in supporting the sustainability of groups over time.

Specific Issues for Substance-Abuse-Related Groups

In recent years, some concerns have arisen about placing high-risk students together in peer groups. The primary concern is that high-risk students can teach deviant behavior to, and reinforce it in, each other. For example, Dishion, McCord, and Poulin (1999) found that in some of their peer-group-based prevention studies, middle school students who received the intervention had worse outcomes on some measures (e.g., tobacco use and teacher-identified problem behavior) than students who did not receive the intervention. Based on these findings, Dishion and his colleagues have warned of the potential for what they call "deviancy training" when high-risk students are grouped together for intervention.

We mention these findings here because group leaders should consider the possibility that students in their substance-abuse-related groups may learn inappropriate behaviors from other group members. One such behavior is telling "war stories" (i.e., stories about their past that glamorize prior drug use). School mental health professionals should be vigilant about addressing this and other inappropriate member behaviors, and should make efforts to redirect such behaviors into something more positive.

The types of negative effects found by Dishion and his colleagues for middle school students have not been found in adolescent substance abuse treatment studies (see Dennis et al., 2004; Waldron & Kaminer, 2004) or in prevention studies for older adolescents (see Eggert, Thompson, Herting, & Randall, 2001). At present, we suggest that the potential for deviancy training can be minimized by providing high-risk students with clearly structured group interventions, as well as with a leader who has the skills to facilitate such a group of students effectively. In addition, any leader should consider the composition of the group during the pregroup interview process, as some potential members may not be appropriate for a peer group intervention.

CASE EXAMPLE

Tamara Clarke had been a school counselor in the Alpine School District for 5 years, working in two elementary schools. She was recently asked to change placements and join Jackson High School to support the guidance counselors and help provide more mental health services to the students. Since her internship and many of her practicum placements during her training had been in high school settings, she was excited about the reassignment. Because the school administrators were seeing a rise in the number of students who were using or experimenting with drugs, they requested the school counselors to focus on drug prevention, as well as to lead groups for students who had received treatment in community settings and were making the transition back to the school setting.

Although Tamara had received training in group counseling and substance abuse, she had never actually led her own support group for students with substance abuse problems, as there was no need for this type of group in her previous work at the elementary school level. Although she was being pressured by the administration to provide such groups, she wanted to make sure she received more training and experience before leading her own group. Accordingly, Tamara spoke with one of the other counselors in the district, Jan Edmunds, who had been running substance abuse support groups in a high school across town. Jan mentioned that she was starting such a group within the next month and suggested that they co-lead the group as a way to provide Tamara with additional training and experience. Tamara spoke with the administrators at Jackson High to provide them with her plan to receive further training before leading her own group. The administrators were supportive, as they had seen previous counselors lead groups without experience, and this had resulted in some very negative feedback from students and parents.

To provide Tamara with an idea of how to set up the group, Jan shared the steps she went through before the first meeting of any group. She first shared the confidentiality forms that she had parents and students sign prior to the first meeting. She stated that she sometimes had a hard time getting parents in to meet with her; if a face-to-face meeting was not possible, she would speak with parents on the phone and would send the confidentiality forms to the home for them to sign. She also provided Tamara with a copy of the pregroup interview questions that she asked each student. Finally, she shared with Tamara her group plan. This allowed Tamara to understand the importance of creating a purpose for the group and setting group goals; it also encouraged her to think about logistical issues that she had not considered before (e.g., ways to do rotating scheduling). One of the main things Tamara had not thought about was the use of various measures before the start of the group and after its ending, in order to collect outcome data on the group. Jan shared with her parent, teacher, and student satisfaction questionnaires, as well as a data sheet she used to keep track of relapses and other outcome measures (such as group attendance and grades).

After providing all of the information about setting up a group, Jan shared the group schedule with Tamara, and they agreed to meet 30 minutes before each group session to go over goals for the session and make sure they were "on the same page." They also agreed to take some time after each session to discuss how it went, what would be done in the next session, and how to improve communication between the two of them and the group members.

Co-leading the group with Jan provided Tamara with the experience and confidence she needed to run her own substance abuse support group. She was able to co-lead the group effectively, but she also learned from Jan ways to handle difficult issues. She learned more about the group process, as well as issues specific to substance abuse and ways to manage and work with resistant members. In particular, two members of the group were there involuntarily and were required to attend in order to continue to play sports at their high school.

One of the things that Tamara noticed while co-leading the group was the difference in responsiveness by Ricardo, a student from a Hispanic (Mexican) background. Tamara mentioned to Jan after the third session that it seemed as if they were not "reaching" him, and that he did not seem to "gel" with the rest of the group. Tamara was particularly concerned, as Jackson High School had a large percentage of Mexican students, and thus many of the members of her group were likely to be Mexican. Jan and Tamara brainstormed ways to encourage more involvement and participation from Ricardo. They read more about Ricardo's culture; they spoke with some of his teachers who were also Mexican and had developed a positive relationship with him; and they met with Ricardo individually to see whether anything could be done to help him get more out of the group. Over the course of the next few group sessions, Jan and Tamara noticed that Ricardo was participating more and sharing more about his family, background, and struggle to maintain abstinence.

At the end of 12 weeks, the group members made a plan to meet monthly to check in and help maintain the progress they had made. Tamara committed to attending these meetings, but was also ready to start her own group at Jackson High. She continued to learn more about the Mexican culture and attended workshops on group processes to further develop her skills as a leader. Within her first year at Jackson High, she ran one 12-

week group with eight students and received feedback from parents, teachers, and students that the group had been beneficial. She also received praise from the administrators, who were pleased to see the progress students had made and to see the counselor take on more of the mental health role for the school.

CHAPTER SUMMARY

Groups are frequently used in school settings, because they are an efficient and effective way for school mental health professionals to serve many students. Psychoeducational and support groups are most appropriate for use in school settings where student substance use and abuse are concerns. Self-help and therapy groups are more appropriate for use in community settings and are frequent components of substance abuse treatment for adolescents. Groups develop over a series of stages that are influenced by such factors as the groups' structure, duration, and purpose. School professionals should develop skills in specific areas in order to facilitate effective groups; some of these areas include basic communication skills, working with resistant members, and cultural awareness/competence. In addition, school professionals must consider many practical aspects of conducting groups, such as scheduling, space, and member attendance. A case example has illustrated how a school counselor obtained the training she needed for conducting groups in her school.

CHAPTER RESOURCES

Resources for Group Manuals and Curricula

National Institute on Alcohol Abuse and Alcoholism (NIAAA)
www.niaaa.nih.gov

The *Cognitive-Behavioral Coping Skills Therapy Manual* (Kadden et al., 1995) can be obtained through this website for a nominal cost. It was originally developed for treating adults with alcohol problems, but has been adapted for adolescents in some research studies. Group leaders can adapt the manual (or components of it) as needed for students. It contains many good modules on coping and skill building.

National Clearinghouse for Alcohol and Drug Information (NCADI)
ncadi.samhsa.gov

Several useful materials are available free of charge through this website: the Cannabis Youth Treatment (CYT) Series, a set of manuals originally developed for a large-scale research project with adolescents (see Chapter 5 for more information about this project); and *Substance Abuse Treatment: Group Therapy* (Treatment Improvement Protocol [TIP] Series 41), an overview of group treatment for substance abuse that is not specifically focused on adolescents but is a good resource in general.

Chestnut Health Systems/Lighthouse Institute
www.chestnut.org/LI/APSS/CSAT/protocols

This website is the source for various treatment manuals that were primarily developed for large federally funded research studies on substance abuse. In particular, there is a group-based manual available under "Adolescent Treatment Models" that can be obtained for a nominal price. This site also provides an overview of many different types of treatment manuals.

Motivational Interviewing Resources

Motivational Interviewing
www.motivationalinterview.org

This is the official website of motivational interviewing and contains much useful information, including where to obtain training, as well as comments from the developers.

Other materials on motivational interviewing are available through the NIAAA and NCADI websites listed above:

- The *Motivational Enhancement Therapy Manual* (Miller, Zweben, DiClemente, & Rychtarik, 1994) is available through the NIAAA site. It was originally developed for adults with alcohol problems, but it (or components of it) can be adapted as needed for students.
- *Enhancing Motivation for Change in Substance Abuse Treatment* (Center for Substance Abuse Treatment, 1999a) is available through the NCADI site. It includes information on the theoretical and practical aspects of motivational interviewing, and contains many good forms and instruments related to the practice of motivational interviewing.
- The CYT Series (see above), also available through the NCADI site, includes modules on motivational interviewing and motivational enhancement therapy that have been adapted for adolescents.

Cultural Diversity Resources

American Psychological Association
www.apa.org

This organization has put together a comprehensive set of guidelines, titled *Guidelines on Multicultural Education, Training, Research, Practice, and Organizational Change for Psychologists*. This document provides much good information and many resources. It can be adapted by school mental health professionals for use in schools.

Other Professional Organizations

(search the Web for URLs)

Most of the professional organizations for school mental health professionals (e.g., school psychologists, school counselors) have developed guidelines in regard to multicultural competency. Go to your organization's website for this information.

K–12 Real Life Issues Curriculum Infusion
www.neiu.edu/~k12pac/index.htm

This website is hosted by Northeastern Illinois University and was developed to help preservice and in-service teachers infuse real-life issues (e.g., substance abuse, bullying, violence) into their curricula. It has some good resources on diversity-related topics that can be adapted by school mental health professionals.

There are also many good books and articles on the topics of diversity and multicultural issues, some of which have been cited in this chapter (e.g., Ivey & Ivey, 2003; Sue et al., 1998). Again, we encourage you to search your professional organization's website for more materials on these topics.

7

Consultation and Referral

CLAUDIA G. VINCENT

Given the scarce resources with which most schools have to operate, and the complexity of substance abuse and its related problems, consultation with community agencies and referral to non-school-based mental health professionals are often necessary. This chapter offers a brief overview of the critical conceptual features of the consultation and referral process; outlines the practical steps of the process; provides guidance on how to negotiate financial responsibilities; offers suggestions on how to build and maintain an effective and efficient referral system; and presents a case example to illustrate the process. A list of resources at the end of the chapter will help readers locate additional information of particular interest to them.

Adequately addressing substance abuse and related problems with school-based resources alone can be a challenge for a variety of reasons. Behaviors related to substance abuse may often be triggered by events or circumstances indirectly related to the school environment, and therefore may be beyond the immediate reach of school personnel. Family dynamics, neighborhood characteristics, and peer groups are powerful influences in students' lives, especially as students reach the age when they begin to question adult expectations, experiment with different lifestyles, and tend to value peer acceptance over teacher or parent approval (Burrow-Sanchez, 2006; Burrow-Sanchez & Lopez, in press; Sales, 2004; Wood, 2003). As they try to define their place within society, adolescent students are particularly vulnerable to social pressures both inside and outside school, and often cannot accurately judge the long-term impact of these influences.

Claudia G. Vincent, PhD, is an administrative assistant in the College of Education at the University of Oregon.

Because school-based help to address problems with substance abuse may often be limited, it becomes necessary under these circumstances to reach out to the community to provide a comprehensive support system for students that spans school, home, and community settings. Community-based services offer a number of advantages over school-based services, including additional time to address the substance abuse, highly focused substance abuse expertise, different settings to provide treatment, and the availability of varying levels of treatment (Adelman & Taylor, 2000; Sales, 2004; Stevens & Morral, 2003). School, home, and community need to develop close collaborations to (1) identify students who are engaging in substance abuse, (2) provide prompt and adequate treatment, and (3) encourage students to seek help by eliminating the social stigma attached to undergoing treatment.

As mental health professionals working in schools, school counselors or psychologists are in pivotal positions to build linkages across settings and service providers. The school counselor or psychologist, who is often the first point of contact when problems with substance abuse arise, can function as a liaison between school and community once school-based service options have been exhausted and additional services are necessary (Burrow-Sanchez & Lopez, in press). To do so effectively and efficiently, the school counselor or psychologist—in collaboration with other school personnel, students, parents, and community mental health professionals—can shape a continuum of services that, although not located on school grounds, are readily and easily available to students who may need them. Collaborations with community agencies may also encourage a sense of shared responsibility among parents, school, and community members for helping students who are engaging in substance abuse.

OVERVIEW OF THE KEY FEATURES OF THE CONSULTATION AND REFERRAL PROCESS

The mental health field has defined a number of models for delivering comprehensive care to individuals for an array of problem behaviors. For example, *systems of care* (Duchnowsky & Kutash, 2005) are carefully coordinated service delivery models that can address multiple needs of individuals and families, reduce costs by eliminating redundant service components, and facilitate access to initial help as well as follow-up care. Similarly, the *wraparound approach* (Eber, Sugai, Smith, & Scott, 2002) addresses the many aspects of an individual's needs and focuses on seamless, effective, and efficient delivery of available services. Adolescents with substance abuse problems may experience—in addition to varying degrees of physical dependence—emotional and behavioral disorders, low academic achievement, family members with medical or mental health problems, or abusive relationships. To provide support for a student with substance abuse and related issues, several community and/or county services may have to be carefully coordinated so that the student benefits. This coordination may range from simple logistics (providing transportation among service providers, arranging for in-home visits) to locating service deliverers with matching philosophies (e.g., strength-based approaches), minimizing redundant eligibility evaluations and paperwork, and establishing consistent expectations across agencies. These comprehensive and efficient service delivery models share a number of critical features, which can be applied to developing a framework for establishing collaborations among school, home, and community to support students with substance abuse problems. To establish an effective, efficient, relevant, and durable network of services beyond the school environment, the consultation and referral process should be all of the following:

1. *Collaborative.* A student's behavior is influenced by multiple factors, all of which need to be considered to shape an intervention that is most likely to be effective. Different individuals (e.g., teachers, school psychologist, school counselor, parents, friends, and relatives) are familiar with different aspects of a student's life; they can offer critical information about events that may be contributing to the student's substance abuse, and that may need to be addressed to design an effective intervention.

2. *Person-centered.* The welfare of the student always comes first. Consultation and referral should never lose sight of the individual student's behaviors and circumstances. Collaboration with family members and consultation with community agencies and service providers can build a system of support that addresses specific needs under specific circumstances. To increase the likelihood that students will complete treatment, the students themselves should play an integral role in defining the best treatment option (Lambie & Rokutani, 2002; Wood, 2003).

3. *Strength-based.* Students with substance abuse problems are more likely to enroll in and complete support programs if service providers recognize, appreciate, and build on the students' personal strengths, talents, and abilities (Eber et al., 2002). A strength-based approach to service delivery can mitigate adversarial feelings between family members or between a student and school personnel that are counterproductive to the student's success.

4. *Culturally sensitive and culturally relevant.* Students' culture influences their behavior and attitudes toward legal and illegal substances. Interventions are most effective if they recognize and value students' and their families' values, attitudes, beliefs, language, religion, economic standing, and other unique characteristics. Sensitivity to students' culture increases the relevance of support, and thus the likelihood that students will take advantage of the services offered and benefit from them.

5. *Data-driven.* Treatment selection and monitoring should always be based on data reflecting students' behaviors of concern. Students who engage in substance abuse are likely to downplay or hide their behavior to avoid unwanted adult attention. To gain an accurate understanding of the severity of a student's problem prior to treatment selection, school personnel need to rely on (1) school records, such as frequency and type of office discipline referrals (e.g., tardiness, truancy, possession or use of substances) or sudden changes in academic performance incongruent with academic ability; (2) police records (e.g., charges of being a minor in possession, public intoxication, or driving while

intoxicated); or (3) if accessible, medical records providing information about medical conditions or prior participation in treatment programs. During treatment, data should be collected regularly to assess the student's progress in the treatment program.

6. *Outcome-oriented.* To increase the school's accountability to its students and their families, consultation and referral should focus on treatment outcomes that are important for each student. A student's success, documented through behavioral and/or academic records, must be the ultimate goal of the process. Identifying the conceptual approach or service delivery model most likely to produce successful student outcomes should be the primary concern.

7. *Systemic.* Although each student's needs are different, the referral process should be guided by clearly defined procedures and policies to facilitate interagency (e.g., treatment provider, school, home) communication, action, follow-up, and emergency responses if necessary. If responsive systems are in place, service delivery can be prompt and efficient.

These general features provide an overall framework for establishing a support network beyond the immediate school environment. Implementing a comprehensive support network requires a number of practical considerations, given the limited personnel time and resources in schools today.

PRACTICAL STEPS FOR NON-SCHOOL-BASED SERVICE DELIVERY

This section provides a step-by-step guide through the consultation and referral process: identifying student needs that exceed the capacity of school-based personnel; gathering critical pieces of information to shape an action plan; locating available resources; and matching those resources to a student's individual needs.

Identifying the Need for Community-Based Services

It is important to note that typical training programs for school professionals include little emphasis on substance abuse. For example, Burrow-Sanchez and Lopez (in press) surveyed a national sample of 289 high school counselors to find out the extent of training received, perceived training needs, and most commonly abused substances. Results indicated that the majority of these high school counselors (1) felt insufficiently prepared to address student substance abuse effectively, due to a lack of preservice training (50% did not take a course in substance abuse) and in-service opportunities to learn about substance abuse; (2) identified screening and assessment, as well as individual interventions, as areas in which they would welcome training; and (3) listed alcohol, marijuana, and cigarettes as the substances most commonly abused by students. A survey of a national sample of 283 middle school counselors provided similar results (Burrow-Sanchez, Lopez, & Slagle, in press). These counselors felt similarly unprepared to respond to students' needs related to substance abuse; they also identified screening and assessment, as well as individual interventions, as primary areas in which they would welcome further training. Of the middle school counselors who indicated that their school had a prevention or intervention program in place, many were unsure of its effectiveness. This seems to indicate the need for regular evaluation of existing programs and dissemination of evaluation results to all school personnel, students, and parents to increase knowledge of effective prevention and intervention strategies. These gaps in the training of school professionals make collaboration with community agencies all the more necessary, to provide students with substance abuse problems the help they need.

Given these circumstances, when does it become advisable for school mental health professionals to seek help from community-based agencies in supporting students with substance abuse issues? Four circumstances come to mind: (1) The school personnel's workload makes it impossible to provide the time necessary to address the students' problems; (2) school-based expertise is too limited to address the severity of the students' problems; (3) school-based services do not produce the desired outcomes; and/or (4) teachers, parents, peers, or the students themselves ask for specialized help that exceeds the school's capacity.

Workload and Availability

The responsibilities of school mental health professionals range from providing help with personal development to guiding career choices to addressing concerns about bullying behaviors to counseling students with substance abuse problems. School psychologists and counselors may have large caseloads spread out over multiple schools, and life skill counselors and mental health aides may serve as case managers responsible for many individuals with varying problems. This wide array of responsibilities, paired often with an enormous and fragmented caseload, can severely tax the ability of school mental health professionals to devote the time and resources needed to the concerns of students struggling with substance abuse.[1]

Although school mental health professionals struggle to allocate their time carefully among too many students and responsibilities, the number of students requiring special attention rises steadily. After a decade of stability, rates of substance abuse among the general school-age population have been rising again since the 1990s (Burrow-Sanchez & Lopez, in press; Wood, 2003). Students with disabilities face an even greater risk than the general population of developing substance abuse problems, because of additional medical conditions, prescription medication, social isolation, or behavioral problems. Among the Individuals with Disabilities Education Act (IDEA) disability categories, students identified with emotional and behavioral disorders face the highest risk of developing

---

[1]During the 2002–2003 school year, the student-to-counselor ratio in the United States varied from 225:1 in Wyoming to 951:1 in California, with a national average of 478:1 (*www.schoolcounselor.org*, retrieved on December 15, 2005). This average ratio far exceeds the 250:1 ratio recommended by the American School Counselor Association, and it demonstrates that the vast majority of school counselors have an excessive workload, which limits their availability for students needing special attention.

substance abuse problems because of unhealthy peer relationships, stressful family environments, or repeated school failure (McCombs & Moore, 2002).[2]

These trends indicate that school mental health professionals face not only excessive workloads, but also complex situations that require highly specialized expertise in divergent areas. Students with an array of problems including substance abuse are likely to require intensive and carefully coordinated services to address their needs. When school-based services do not have the capacity to address all of a student's needs, community agencies may be able to provide needed assistance. Rather than fitting the student *into* school-based services, providers need to fit available services *around* the student, who remains at the center of the consultation and referral process.

Severity of the Problem

Substance abuse and related behaviors present complex problems and require expertise with a variety of mental health issues, including physical dependence, complicated family histories, and negative peer relationships. Given the wide array of responsibilities of school mental health professionals, it is unrealistic to expect them to be knowledgeable about all aspects of these behaviors and be able to provide services geared specifically toward addressing them. Community-based services are much more likely to provide the specialized knowledge necessary to shape an effective intervention for a specific problem. Because a student's welfare is the ultimate concern of school personnel, community assistance should be recruited when the student's needs exceed school-based expertise (Burrow-Sanchez & Lopez, in press).

Cases Where School-Based Services Do Not Lead to Desired Outcomes

Because of excessive workloads and the complexity of substance abuse and related behaviors, school-based services, even though carefully planned and implemented with fidelity, may not lead to the desired outcomes. To assess whether the school-based services are adequate for a student's needs, clear expectations of changes in the students' behavior need to be formulated, and data should be collected to determine if the expectations are met within a clearly defined time frame. For example, if a student is known to experiment with illegal drugs, steps to decrease his or her risk behavior should be defined, and the frequency of his or her drug use should be carefully monitored to determine whether the intervention is effective. Unfortunately, reliable data on a student's drug use may be difficult to collect, especially when drug use occurs primarily off campus. Student self-

---

[2]Within the general school-age population, 6.2% of students meet the diagnostic criteria for substance abuse as a disorder. Special populations, however, have far higher prevalence rates: 62.1% of students involved with the juvenile justice system, 19.2% of students involved with child welfare, 40.8% of students with mental health issues, and 23.6% of students with serious emotional disorders meet the diagnostic criteria for substance abuse (Wood, 2003).

reports, or reports from peers and family members, may provide some indication of the intervention's effect. If such data indicate that the counseling services offered through the school do not result in the expected behavioral changes within the defined time frame, referral to community-based services should be considered. An outside referral does not mean that the school is no longer responsible for the student's welfare; it simply means that the school reaches out to the community to provide a more extensive support network (Adelman & Taylor, 1997, 2000; Knudson, Kamara, & Louden, 1992).

Requests from Teachers, Parents, Peers, or Students for Additional Help

The most direct indicators that referral to community agencies is necessary are concerned individuals asking for help the school is unable to provide. The following are signs that additional help may be necessary: (1) Teachers may become aware that a student's behavior is not changing favorably or that his or her academic performance continues to deteriorate; (2) parents may notice changes in their child's behaviors, interests, interactions with others, or emotional accessibility; (3) peers may be concerned about a friend's changing activity patterns; or (4) a student currently receiving school services might indicate that his or her needs are not entirely met. For example, a 10th-grade English teacher notices that Susan, who has had several office discipline referrals for smoking marijuana in the school bathrooms and has received school-based counseling for drug use, attends his class only sporadically and is unprepared and withdrawn when she does. During a parent conference, Susan's father confirms that in spite of the counseling services Susan receives at school, her withdrawal from family and school life has increased. Worried about his daughter's future and her nonresponsiveness to the school's counseling services, the father asks for an appointment with the school counselor to discuss changes in intervention strategies, including referral to community-based services.

All members of the school community should feel comfortable about requesting additional help. Open communication is essential to shape interventions that lead to desired outcomes. An atmosphere of mutual trust among students, teachers, parents, and school personnel encourages all members of the school community to take responsibility for each other and voice concerns. Information exchange is critical to building a comprehensive and seamless support network that spans multiple environments and situations, and that can give students access to necessary resources.

Teachers, parents, and peers are knowledgeable about very different aspects of a student's life. This diversity of perspectives is helpful to identify approaches that address all aspects of students' needs, are sensitive to their culture, and therefore are more likely to be perceived as relevant and worthwhile by their families. The target students themselves are invaluable sources of information. Depending on their level of maturity and the extent to which they acknowledge their problems, they may be instrumental in shaping interventions that are of greatest benefit to them.

Finally, it is also important to keep in mind that schools are not required by law to provide interventions for substance abuse. Although a student's substance abuse problem is primarily the responsibility of the parents, schools can play an important role in assisting parents to locate needed help and assure that the treatment is appropriate and effective.

In summary, because students with substance abuse problems have intense and complex needs and because schools have limited resources, consultation with and referral to community services becomes necessary when one or more of the following are true:

1. A student's problems cannot be adequately addressed within the available schedules of school mental health professionals.
2. The severity of the student's problem requires specialized or comprehensive care.
3. School-based services do not lead to improved behavior within the expected time frame.
4. Concerned individuals request additional help.

Once the need for non-school-based services has been clearly identified, school mental health professionals can play important roles in providing the student with efficient and effective access to community-based services. The following section offers guidelines to make this process collaborative, person-centered, strength-based, culturally sensitive and relevant, data-driven, and outcome-oriented.

Gathering Critical Pieces of Information to Shape an Action Plan

To assure effective and efficient implementation of an intervention and coordination across settings, it is useful to develop an action plan. This collaboratively developed written document specifies the intervention strategy, the steps of the implementation process, individual responsibilities, and monitoring procedures. It represents a crucial step in moving from identified needs and potential strategies for addressing those needs to specific actions.

When a student with substance abuse problems would benefit from community services, an action plan can be a useful tool to establish continuity between school and community to facilitate the student's seamless access to needed help, avoid redundancies in services, promote a sense of shared responsibility, and limit disruption of the student's school and home life. To achieve these goals, school mental health professionals can actively solicit the collaboration of teachers, students, parents, and peers. Data-based assessments of a student's changes in behavior provide focus and relevance to the collaboration.

Soliciting Collaboration of Teachers, Students, Parents, and Peers

Informal and formal networking efforts can raise schoolwide and communitywide awareness of the problems some students face, and can mobilize community resources to prevent or offer help to address those problems. To build successful collaborations and effective partnerships among school constituencies and across agencies, several issues are critical: (1) an atmosphere of mutual trust where open and honest communication can occur; (2) a person-centered focus; (3) adherence to confidentiality requirements; and (4) ongoing communication between school and community agencies.

MUTUAL TRUST

Without open and honest communication, identification of potentially severe problems and prompt responses to those problems are extremely difficult. All school personnel need to collaborate seamlessly to develop a system of support that addresses all aspects of a student's problem behavior. Keeping in mind that the student's welfare always comes first, each individual participating in the information-gathering process needs to suspend his or her personal interests and focus exclusively on the student.

To start working toward developing an action plan, the school mental health professional should consult with as many sources as necessary, including teachers who know the student well, administrative staff, parents and family members, peers, and close friends. Most importantly, the student in need of support should be an integral element of this consultation process (see "Person-Centered Focus," below). The school mental health professional's unique position as liaison among multiple individuals who know the student well allows him or her to create a comprehensive profile of the student's behavior, so that all involved share an awareness of the complexity and scope of the problem.

The school mental health professional should approach each potential source of information with an understanding of his or her relationship to the student. Sensitivity, efficiency, and comprehensiveness should drive the consultation process, so that the resulting action plan precisely targets the specific characteristics of the student's substance abuse. All participants in the process need to understand that substance abuse has multiple causes and that no one person is solely responsible for the student's behavior. Parents may feel placed in an awkward position if there is a family history of substance abuse. However, a focus on the student's and his or her family's strengths and future can put the process into a positive context and prevent potential scapegoating.

PERSON-CENTERED FOCUS

As indicated above, the most important source of information is the student with substance abuse problems him- or herself. The person-centered focus of the consultation and referral process puts the student at the center of all service planning and delivery. The student's contributions to the consultation process are likely to vary with his or her age and maturity level. Depending on the student's attitude toward drug use, the family's potential denial of the problem, and fear of legal ramifications, there may be significant resistance to receiving treatment. To minimize such resistance, it is important to give the student an active voice in shaping an action plan. Research indicates that students rate prevention and treatment approaches that include hands-on activities (e.g., visiting treatment facilities, interviewing facility personnel, developing and distributing posters displaying prevention messages) as more relevant than programs that simply tell the students what to do or not to do without allowing for student input (Wood, 2003). If the student considers the services irrelevant, experiences the delivery settings as aversive and uncomfortable, or feels excluded from the decision-making process, he or she is unlikely to follow through with the intervention (Lambie & Rokutani, 2002). To facilitate the student's inclusion and active participation, care should be taken to include individuals who share the student's culture and can relate to his or her individual circumstances. These strategies are likely to increase the comfort level for the student and for any family members who might perceive the school environment as alienating.

Unless the student declines, initial consultation meetings between school personnel and parents should include the student as an active contributor to the process of shaping an intervention that will lead to desired outcomes. Since the student is at the center of the discussion, and his or her well-being is the very reason for the meeting, he or she represents the best source of information. Depending on the student's maturity and willingness, he or she could facilitate the meeting by preparing a set of questions or discussion items, or—at a minimum—could be asked for guidance on what would assist him or her to make changes in behavior. Parents and school mental health professionals should also make certain that the student understands all features of a treatment option, has time to reflect and consider options, and is encouraged to ask questions.

If the student feels uncomfortable speaking up at meetings, he or she could prepare materials prior to the meeting and ask an adult to present them to the group. For example, the student could compose a chart depicting his or her goals for the future and what he or she perceives as potential barriers in reaching those goals. Or the student might write a short story that might help others understand the reasons for his or her behaviors. It is important to approach the problem from the perspective of the individual student, to integrate his or her voice in the planning process, and to focus on the student's strengths in order to identify an intervention that is likely to be successful for him or her.

CONFIDENTIALITY

When soliciting information from a number of individuals, the school mental health professional needs to be careful not to violate confidentiality policies. Confidentiality requirements are governed by district and agency policies as well as legal mandates. School mental health professionals must abide by Title 42 of the U.S. Code of Federal Regulations, Part 2 (42 CFR), which regulates "the confidentiality of AOD [alcohol and other drug] abuse patient records" (Fisher & Harrison, 2005, p. 322). Application of the regulations requires a good deal of interpretation and judgment, particularly within a collaborative approach where individuals contributing information and services may operate under different sets of policies. In general, all information regarding substance use and abuse must be treated with the utmost confidentiality; this means that the school mental health professional should not share identifying information with individuals not immediately involved with the student's treatment. When necessary, written consent to disclose information to those involved in developing the required support network can be requested to assure compliance with federal regulations. In the case of a minor student, state law may require parental consent before treatment at a community agency can begin. Because legal mandates vary from state to state, it is best to seek legal counsel if there are questions about how to handle disclosure of information (Fisher & Harrison, 2005). Please see Chapter 1 for more detailed information related to confidentiality.

COMMUNICATION ACROSS AGENCIES

A balance between open communication and adherence to confidentiality requirements should define communications among school personnel, families, and community agencies. Seamless support, minimal redundancy of services, and maximal benefit of interventions depend on regular and ongoing information exchange among all individuals providing services to a student. The school mental health professional can take the lead in setting up a communication schedule that assures continuity across sites and promotes ongoing shared responsibility for the student's treatment success. For example, those involved in developing and monitoring the student's treatment should be able to meet at regular intervals to review progress data and assess the need for changes in the treatment. At the beginning of a treatment program, weekly or biweekly meetings may be necessary to assure that the student attends treatment sessions and receives an intervention that meets his or her needs. As the treatment progresses, meetings may occur less often. In addition, parents, treatment providers, and school personnel should exchange contact information (phone numbers, email addresses) in case unscheduled emergency contact is necessary.

Documentation of the Student's Needs

During the informal and formal information-gathering process, documentation of the student's needs provides direction and relevance, and keeps participants committed to the student's success. Documentation of student needs may also be required for federal and local accountability standards.

Data gathered during the initial phase provide a baseline for assessing the student's responsiveness to the intervention once treatment begins. Given the complexity and often covert nature of substance abuse and related behaviors, establishing a reliable data record can be challenging. Information from multiple sources in the form of completed questionnaires, discipline referrals, teacher and parent reports, or self-reports can contribute to documenting a student's needs. To increase the usefulness of data, they should be collected regularly, with reliable and valid measures; they might include times of day and locations when the student is most likely to engage in risky behaviors, as well as frequency of drug use or concomitant behaviors of concern (such as lying, truancy, or decreases in academic performance). A checklist completed by the school mental health professional might be a useful tool to determine whether (1) data collection occurs regularly, (2) the student makes or fails to make progress toward established goals, and (3) the intervention needs to be adjusted to be more effective. Chapters 3 and 5 provide more detailed information on screening, assessment, and data collection.

Once the student receives services through a community-based agency, the data collection system must be responsive to interagency use. School and agency personnel should agree on the method and frequency of data collection, and on what data will be most useful. Community mental health providers have their own record-keeping systems, which are likely protected against disclosure under 42 CFR. If data cannot be shared, the school can try to negotiate additional data collection with the agency to establish records that are accessible to school as well as agency personnel.

Consultants and service providers are likely to collect data regularly only if the data are actively used for decision making. All individuals participating in shaping a support network for the student will appreciate seeing the student's needs and progress clearly documented. For example, a clearly visible trend toward improved academic performance (documented by how many assignments the student completed and what grades he or she received), or fewer office discipline referrals for drug use, can illustrate progress and be reason for celebration.

In aggregated form without identifying information, the entire school community might benefit from learning about risk indicators and treatment approaches. For example, a school might develop a summary of student risk behaviors (e.g., truancy, use of different substances, social withdrawal), the frequency with which they occur at the school, local levels of reported substance use, and available school-based and community-based treatment options. This summary could be posted in the teen health education classroom, or made available to students and parents via handouts or newsletters. If the school regularly asks students to assess their school's climate (including protective factors, such as positive peer relations and positive student–teacher relations), these survey results could also be posted in the school or disseminated via newsletter. Appropriately used, these data can become teaching tools and raise students', teachers', and parents' awareness of the warning signs indicating emerging problems and available treatment options in the community.

Additional Considerations

Although a student's immediate and long-term mental health should drive the consultation process and the referral decision, it is equally important to select treatment programs that are responsive to the student's and his or her family's cultural background and individual circumstances and expectations. A student is more likely to follow a treatment plan that takes into consideration his or her own and the family's unique characteristics and needs. These unique features range from ethnicity, language, disability status, and gender to socioeconomic status (SES) and belief systems. Some individual features may require careful coordination of multiple services; others (e.g., transportation needs for low-SES families) may be more easily addressed. The following sections provide broad guidelines for addressing particular individual needs to maximize the likelihood that the student will follow through with a referral and benefit from appropriate treatment. Because each school has its own demographic characteristics, culturally sensitive practices will differ according to the school's population. Each of the guidelines below should be interpreted in the context of a school's specific culture and demographics, as well as the context of the individual student's culture.

CULTURAL SENSITIVITY AND RELEVANCE

Any treatment's success depends in some measure on the student's comfort with the treatment provider. Although concerns about health risks are primary, all individuals involved in the treatment selection and implementation process must be aware of cultural differences that could impede a student's adherence to a treatment plan. Cultural characteristics of treatment provider and recipient, including language, ethnicity, and belief system, need to be carefully considered for maximum success of the identified treatment option (Sheridan, 2000). In his or her capacity of liaison among a student, family, and community agency, the school mental health professional can encourage awareness of individual differences, help participants to articulate underlying assumptions or discomforts without fear of repercussions, and assist in identifying strategies to address those differences in a constructive manner. For example, an Asian American female student who has been given multiple office discipline referrals for using alcohol on campus by the European American male principal of her school might feel antagonistic toward a European American male treatment provider. However, if these feelings are openly discussed, perhaps either discomfort can be overcome, or the student can be reassigned to a provider with whom she feels more comfortable. Sporadic checks during treatment regarding overall satisfaction with treatment delivery and progress might be a strategy to maintain good relations between the service provider and the student, and thus to avoid premature termination of treatment.

The school mental health professional can play an important role in addressing cultural differences by actively soliciting feedback from students and family members who need additional help. For example, a questionnaire handed out during an initial meeting might ask for a student's and family's preferred language and available means of transportation. It might also ask them to rate their perceptions of social norms or autonomy, and to define their understanding of substance use and their family's norms on this topic. The overall goal is to gather as much information as possible from the student and his or her family, to make sure that the services the student will receive are a good match for his or her needs, and that the student feels comfortable with the service provider.

If language barriers exist, translators and interpreters can assist with communication. The school counselor should have a list of interpreter service providers available. Because it is important for an interpreter to be unbiased, use of family members or interpreters known to the family should be discouraged. The interpreter should be familiar with the basic terminology used during consultation, should be encouraged to ask clarifying questions when necessary, and can provide useful feedback about how to shape the communication process to make it maximally beneficial for the student and his or her family (Turnbull, Turnbull, Shank, & Smith, 2004). It is also important for the interpreter to be familiar with and trained in how to adhere to the legal mandates governing relationships and interactions between school mental health professionals and students, particularly confidentiality regulations.

School mental health professionals who speak only English, but who often work with students and families for whom English is a second language, might consider learning basic phrases in their students' primary language(s) (e.g., "Hello," "How are you?"). This small gesture can help establish a collaborative relationship between school personnel and families, and can increase the comfort level of family members when they consult with school personnel about a child's substance abuse.

RESPECT FOR PRIVACY

Collecting information about individual perceptions and preferences must be carefully balanced with respect for a student's and family's privacy. Although privacy expectations differ among cultural groups, it is important to balance professional accountability requirements, cultural expectations, and the need to collaborate effectively with the need for privacy to minimize potential embarrassment and stigmatizing. All individuals participating in the consultation and referral process need to be instructed to share information only with those who need to know the circumstances of a student's substance abuse and related problems in order to provide professional services. As mentioned earlier, confidentiality regarding substance abuse is regulated by federal legislation (42 CFR). Chapter 1 provides more detailed information about the content and application of 42 CFR.

PARENTAL CONSENT

State law determines whether parental consent is required before a minor student can be referred to a community agency for substance abuse treatment (Fisher & Harrison, 2005). The World Wide Web is a good and easily accessible resource for finding out which treatments require parental consent in which state. Because states differ in their parental consent requirements, it might be best to consult your local school district or state policies. Often both parent and student signatures are required for treatment to begin. If a student initially confides in school personnel instead of his or her parents, a school mental health professional may be obligated to inform the parents of the problem. Before notifying parents, however, school personnel should check local state and district policies regarding confidentiality issues. If such an approach is allowable under local policies, parental notification should occur in a manner that does not penalize the student for seeking help. The school mental health professional can request a formal or informal meeting with the parents to inform them of the problem, as well as to learn about their perspectives on substance abuse and available treatment options. Exact procedures and legal mandates to solicit parental consent need to be determined by the school administrator and school personnel.

Locating Available Resources

Exploring community-based service options typically occurs reactively, after a student has been identified or after data collection indicates that the school's mental health services are inadequate to address the student's immediate and long-term needs. The school mental health professional can then assume a leadership role in locating available and appropriate community resources that address the student's needs. Forging short-term and long-term relationships between school and community through referrals of students to community-based services is an important component of shaping a continuum of service options for students with substance abuse and related problems.

Ideally, however, this step of the process occurs proactively. The overall goal is to assure prompt accessibility of services for students with intense problems. Therefore, the school mental health professional might proactively explore available services and establish connections with community service providers, so that linkages are in place when they are needed. These proactively forged linkages will—by necessity—be generic service options. The school might maintain an up-to-date list with the primary contact information for community agencies providing services ranging from psychoeducation to residential treatments. The school might also furnish each service provider with names and other contact information for its mental health professionals, so that collaborative relationships can be more easily established. Once a specific student has been identified and his or her circumstances documented through the information-gathering process described above, these service providers can be contacted and consulted for an individualized treatment plan. An existing list of service providers with each provider's service capacity can accelerate the design of an individually tailored treatment in collaboration with the student, his or her family, and the school professional to address a specific set of behaviors or concerns in a practical manner.

As a mental health professional familiar with the various constituencies of the school and the local mental health community, the school counselor, psychologist, or intervention specialist is in a position to network with a large number of people from various professional backgrounds. Unstructured networking through conversations with teachers, administrators, parents, colleagues, or friends and acquaintances who share interests, concerns, and experiences might lead toward structured exploration of available services. The World Wide Web provides useful tools in locating services. For example, a website maintained by the Substance Abuse and Mental Health Services Administration (*findtreatment.samhsa.gov*) provides links to a national directory of treatment services. Individual communities that maintain their own locator services can easily be found with Web search engines.

Establishing a structured and easily accessible network of services means building durable partnerships with community service providers. Key features to be considered while exploring potential partnerships include (1) agency capacity, (2) a continuum of services to address varying needs, (3) durability of relationships, and (4) dissemination of information. The overall goal in establishing partnerships is always improving the welfare of students. Thus philosophical and conceptual differences in service design and delivery should not limit the school mental health professional's willingness to approach community service providers for potential collaborations.

Agency Capacity

Seamless transitions from school-based interventions to community-based services, with a minimum of bureaucratic delay and no redundancies in services, are desirable. Because a student's commitment to pursuing treatment may be tentative, undue delays and obstacles are likely to jeopardize successful treatment implementation. Above all, any agency suitable to provide services to middle or high school students should be experienced with treating adolescents. Adolescents have very specific needs, including a strong desire for autonomous decision making and resistance to adult authority (Lambie & Rokutani, 2002). Treatment approaches should take these needs into consideration. Interactive programs allowing students to be active participants in their treatment have been rated as more successful by both students and researchers (Wood, 2003). In addition to adolescent-focused approaches, the agency should have the capacity to address the needs of varying cultural groups, be willing to negotiate payment responsibilities with parents or guardians, and be interested in a long-term partnership.

Continuum of Treatment Options

A list of available community services should span a continuum of treatment options with varying intensity. Not only students with the most severe and immediate problems may have to be referred to community agencies; students who remain unresponsive to school-based mental health services may also benefit from services available in the community. Students with lasting and complex needs should feel comfortable accessing school and community services alternately or concurrently. Chapters 5 and 6 provide detailed information on individual- and group-based treatment interventions, respectively.

Durability of Relationships

Building durable partnerships to provide a full spectrum of service options requires mutual commitments from school and community agencies. Readiness to enter into such a commitment might be initially explored through phone inquiries or correspondence, and then further nurtured through site visits, workshops, or presentations. The school mental health professional can extend invitations to representatives of community agencies or visit a service provider to gather information and establish professional relationships. Personal contact between service providers will allow exploration of mutual interests and common goals, permit open discussion of needs and capacities, and strengthen commitment to each other (Adelman & Taylor, 1997; Crane & Skinner, 2003; Knudson et al., 1992). Once a partnership has been established, ongoing personal contact can reinforce existing collaborations, keep all partners apprised of changes in services or personnel, introduce new personnel, and provide a forum to discuss concerns and celebrate successes. Ongoing communication is critical to cultivate and sustain a partnership that spans different facilities and clientele.

Dissemination of Information

Once school personnel have mapped out a continuum of available services, this valuable information needs to be disseminated to all members of the school community. The more school personnel, students, teachers, administrators, and parents know about existing service options, the more likely they are to suggest treatment for a student whose behavior is of concern. Widespread knowledge about the existing service continuum also provides clarity about the referral process and establishes continuity between school and community.

Several dissemination strategies can be considered. Printed information is relatively easy to produce and can be posted or otherwise made available in the school, mailed to parents, or included in the school's newsletter. Students might benefit from more direct delivery of information through in-class presentations or workshops. These activities might be incorporated into the school curriculum (e.g., health education classes), might involve both teaching and nonteaching school personnel, and should actively engage students. Students who are familiar with warning signs that might indicate substance abuse problems, and who know about the school's available services and linkages with community agencies, may be more likely to encourage a peer to seek help or to approach an adult with concerns about a peer's behavior. It is important to include the entire student body and their families, as well as general and special education teachers, in these activities; doing so will emphasize the notion that substance abuse can affect everyone and, once it occurs, needs to be openly acknowledged in order to be successfully addressed. Collective support from the school community might encourage a student to acknowledge and seek treatment for substance abuse.

Matching Available Services with a Student's Needs

The complexity of substance abuse and related problems can make finding appropriate treatment for a specific student challenging. A number of issues and considerations should inform the selection of specific services. A treatment option for an individual student should be (1) least disruptive to his or her usual environment and maximally effective to address his or her problem; (2) strength-based and person-centered; (3) able to address multiple coexisting problems, if necessary; (4) include family members, if appropriate; and (5) be culturally responsive (Fisher & Harrison, 2005; Stevens & Morral, 2003).

An array of service delivery options exists, depending on the severity of the student's problem behavior. The following discussion addresses five types of services in order from least intensive to most intensive: (1) psychoeducation, (2) outpatient treatment, (3) day treatment, (4) inpatient treatment, and (5) residential treatment. The advantages and disadvantages of each service delivery model are presented with some selection guidelines. Chapters 5 and 6 provide additional detailed information on specific treatment options. Table 7.1 provides a summary overview of the treatment options available in most communities, their defining features, and their advantages and disadvantages. This overview should be understood as the general case; each treatment program and its application will differ based on individual circumstances.

Psychoeducation

Students who use illegal substances experimentally or recreationally (as documented through high numbers of discipline referrals or other behavioral concerns) and are at risk of developing substance abuse might benefit from psychoeducation. Psychoeducation is a form of early, preventive intervention designed to increase students' awareness and understanding of their behavior, its antecedents, and its potential consequences, as well as to teach strategies that allow the students to avoid negative consequences through self-management. The defining features of self-management strategies are that the students learn (1) to recognize environmental triggers that are likely to result in inappropriate behavior; and (2) to apply strategies including self-control, self-evaluation, and self-reinforcement to neutralize those triggers and thereby avoid inappropriate behavior (Alberto & Troutman, 2003). Depending on the length and intensity of treatment deemed necessary to address an individual student's risk behaviors, psychoeducation could be administered through school-based counseling—possibly as a group intervention—or delivered through a community agency.

To maximize the effectiveness of psychoeducation, intervention delivery should actively engage students in the learning process. For example, with the help of the school counselor or community-based mental health professional, students can learn how to (1) recognize situations that increase the likelihood that they will engage in high-risk behaviors, (2) document their risky behaviors in a variety of environments, and (3) self-administer positive and negative consequences based on clearly defined goals and expectations. Active participation through self-assessment and record keeping enhances students' awareness of their own behavior, its potential risk for themselves and others, and their ability to control and change their behavior. For example, Harry, who had received several office discipline referrals during the last month for smoking cigarettes on campus, was referred to the school counselor. Through an initial consultation, the school counselor found out that Harry smoked to calm his nerves prior to stressful academic situations (tests, difficult assignments) or social situations (contact with others who were likely to tease him). Harry indicated that he would prefer to handle stressful situations differently and was willing to try self-management strategies.

Self-management strategies, including setting goals, self-recording behavior, self-evaluating, and self-reinforcing, give adolescent students who are motivated to change their behavior the opportunity to act autonomously. Setting goals gives the intervention direction and focus. Students should be encouraged to set realistic yet challenging goals. Aiming too high can lead to frustration and discouragement; aiming too low can make the

TABLE 7.1. Overview of Continuum of Services

Continuum of substance use	Continuum of services	Defining features	Advantages	Disadvantages
Risk for abuse (e.g, office discipline referrals related to substance use; sudden drop in academic performance; social withdrawal)	School counseling or other school-based services (such as group-based interventions)	• In-school service • Group-based or individualized	• Nondisruptive of school experience	• Unlimited access to deviant peers
Experimental use (sporadic use, strong affiliation with peers who are using); recreational use (occasional use; risk for abuse	Psychoeducation	• Self-management strategies • School-based or community-based	• Integrated into school day • Low effort • Active student engagement	• Limited effectiveness • Continued contact with deviant peers
Abuse or early dependence (frequent use)	Outpatient	• Community mental health center • 1–16 hours per week	• Continued school attendance • Inclusion of family members	• Continued contact with deviant peer group • Limited supervision
Dependence (regular use)	Day treatment	• Day-long supervision • Individualized treatment plan • Formation of new peer relationships	• Limited access to deviant peer groups • Living at home	• Removal from school • Access to deviant peer group at night
Increasing dependence (regular use, limited motivation to stop using)	Inpatient	• Constant supervision • Access to medical treatment • Short-term isolation from natural environment	• No contact with deviant peer group • Drug abstinence • Teaching of prosocial skills	• Complete removal from natural setting • Limited generalization of skills
Severe dependence (compulsive use; overt physical symptoms—e.g., intoxication, delirium)	Residential	• Constant supervision • Access to detoxification • Isolated setting, rigid schedules	• Isolation from natural environment and social networks • Intense teaching of prosocial skills	• Long-term disruption of school experience and natural development • Risk of dropping out

intervention irrelevant and ineffective. Harry, for example, decided with the help of the school counselor to decrease his smoking by anticipating stressful situations well in advance, thereby decreasing his anxiety. He also agreed to limit his smoking to not more than twice a week for 3 weeks, then to smoke no more than once a week for 2 weeks, and finally to stop entirely. Self-recording behavior will put a student in charge of documenting his or her progress. A variety of methods can be used to record one's own behavior, from simple tally sheets to checklists to elaborate computer programs. Harry was given weekly calendar sheets that contained his class schedule. At the beginning of each week, he recorded all upcoming assignments, tests, and social contacts that he anticipated to be stressful. On the same sheet, he recorded when he smoked. At the end of each week, he tallied the number of stressful events and the number of times he smoked. Summarizing the data at regular intervals allows a student to see his or her progress and share accomplishments with others. Based on his or her documented progress and previously clearly defined goals, the student can self-administer rewards—for example, a preferred activity. After 3 weeks, Harry was able to document that his smoking had decreased to an average of twice a week, and after 4 weeks he recorded no smoking activity at all. To celebrate his success, Harry treated himself to a movie with his best friend.

The advantages of psychoeducation include the active involvement of a student who is showing behaviors of concern and the ease of administering the intervention to a group of students with similar risk behaviors. Potential disadvantages include the possibility that students will not accurately and consistently apply the self-management strategies, thereby making the intervention ineffective. If the intervention is administered to a group of students, there is also a risk that students may learn inappropriate behaviors from each other, jeopardizing the success of the intervention. It is important to keep in mind that psychoeducation is not a treatment, but rather an early, preventive intervention; depending on the severity of a student's substance problem, it might need to be combined with other intervention strategies to change the student's behavior.

Outpatient Treatment

If a student remains unresponsive to psychoeducation, if his or her behaviors indicate frequent use of illegal substances that cannot be adequately addressed through self-management strategies, or if the student exhibits diagnostic criteria for substance abuse or early substance dependence, the school mental health professional may recommend outpatient treatment options available in the community. Outpatient treatment can be group-based, individualized, or both, and often includes the student's family. Its defining features are that the treatment occurs at a community-based mental health center where the student attends counseling sessions from 1 to 16 hours a week. A comprehensive biopsychosocial assessment at intake determines the appropriate treatment intensity. The student is closely monitored throughout treatment and must meet certain exit criteria before discontinuing treatment (Fisher & Harrison, 2005; Stevens & Morral, 2003).

Before referring a student to outpatient treatment, the school mental health professional should consider whether the student is likely to benefit from the treatment. Chapters 3 and 5 provide detailed information on procedures school personnel can use to assess a student's substance abuse. Mental health professionals rely on the placement criteria developed by the American Society of Addiction Medicine (2002) to assess the individual's problem and select a course of treatment appropriate for the severity of the problem. Some considerations for successful outpatient treatment include the individual's (1) motivation to change his or her behavior, (2) physical capability to stop using illicit substances, (3) access to a social support system, (4) family history of substance abuse, and (5) prior treatment history. If the student is likely to benefit from outpatient treatment, the school mental health professional can recommend treatment at a community-based agency with the capacity to offer services that are responsive to the student's individual circumstances. In addition to the considerations listed above, simple logistical concerns (e.g., available transportation or parental participation in the treatment) may be important.

Mental health professionals use a variety of approaches to providing outpatient services based on a variety of theories: behavioral theories (observable behaviors occur in response to an environmental trigger and are maintained by a rewarding consequence); cognitive theories (behavior is regulated by thought processes); social learning theories (behavior is learned via modeling by others); and 12-step programs (recoveries from addictions are based on faith and accomplished through peer support). Some approaches may blend elements of different theories. The conceptual framework used by a specific provider should not be a determining factor, but its match with the student's needs should be. Services that are carefully tailored to the student's needs, are well matched with the family's cultural background and specific circumstances, and have documented effectiveness should be considered.

Among the advantages of outpatient treatment are the student's ability to continue attending school while in treatment, and the treatment's potential inclusion of family members. The disadvantages of outpatient treatment include the student's ability to maintain contact with peer groups that might encourage continued risky behaviors, as well as continued exposure to the environmental situations that have contributed to the substance abuse problem. As the least intensive treatment option, outpatient treatment is suitable for students with early substance dependence, but not for students with established substance dependence. Intensive outpatient treatment offers the option of more frequent counseling sessions at the outpatient facility, which may be necessary, depending on the severity of the student's problem. However, more frequent treatment sessions are also more disruptive to the daily schedules of the student and his or her family.

Day Treatment

On the continuum of treatment options, day treatment should be considered if a student remains unresponsive to outpatient treatment, or if—in the school personnel's judgment—the student (1) has limited motivation to change his or her behavior, (2) is becoming physically dependent on illegal substances, (3) has limited access to a social support system, (4) has a family history of substance abuse, and (5) has not benefited from less intensive treatment. Community-based day treatment options are usually available through treatment centers or hospitals. The defining features of day treatment are that the student spends the majority of his or her day within the treatment setting, and only evenings and nights at home (Fisher & Harrison, 2005). The overall goals of day treatment are to distance the student from activities and contacts with deviant peer groups, teach alternative behaviors, and encourage him or her to form new and constructive peer relationships.

Day treatment usually consists of intensive counseling sessions designed to raise the student's awareness of his or her risk behaviors and their consequences, as well as school or work activities. After referral to a day treatment facility, staff members typically perform a thorough biopsychosocial assessment to determine the most appropriate individualized treatment plan. At the beginning of treatment, students are encouraged to form friendships with others participating in the treatment; this may occur through imposing restrictions on contacts with people who are not treatment participants. During this initial phase, contact with outside peer groups involved in substance abuse is strongly discouraged. Once the student has demonstrated the ability and willingness to follow the treatment facility's behavioral expectations, he or she can expand the social network to include people not participating in treatment, except for previous peers still involved in substance abuse (Stevens & Morral, 2003). Day treatment programs vary in length, depending on the student's progress toward meeting established exit criteria.

The advantages of day treatment are the close supervision of a student's activities and peer contacts during the day, while maintaining contact with his or her family and natural environment by living at home. This combination of intense treatment with regular and predictable contact with the natural environment may facilitate application of new skills and behaviors in nontrained settings as the student expands his or her social network beyond the treatment setting. The student is likely to apply what he or she learns during the day to situations in the natural environment. The major disadvantages of day treatment are that it removes the student from school, disrupts progression through the school curriculum, and potentially stigmatizes the student within the school community. In addition, although the student participates in treatment during the day, he or she may continue to have contact with deviant peers in the evening or at night, and treatment will be less effective if the student continues to engage in risky behaviors when not supervised.

Inpatient Treatment

If the student does not respond to day treatment or relapses into destructive behaviors after day treatment is over, more intense treatment options need to be considered. Inpatient programs offer heightened intensity of treatment for students who have been diagnosed with substance dependence and who might be sufficiently motivated to change their behavior, given the appropriate circumstances. The defining features of inpatient treatment are 24-hour supervision, administration of detoxification services if needed, and short-term isolation from the natural environment. The average duration of inpatient treatments is 28 days (Fisher & Harrison, 2005).

Inpatient treatment, like other mental health services, begins with a comprehensive assessment of the student's medical, psychological, and social needs to design an individualized treatment plan. As in day treatment, the overall goals of inpatient treatment are the formation of a healthy peer group and the acquisition of skills necessary to withstand social pressures to participate in self-destructive behaviors. Depending on the severity of the student's substance dependence, these resocialization activities are combined with a medical detoxification regimen. Abstinence is a prerequisite for participation in treatment activities and therefore constitutes the initial step of most inpatient treatment programs. Once abstinence has been established, treatment usually focuses on developing positive coping skills within the core psychosocial domains of adolescence (i.e., school, family, and peer networks) through counseling sessions and educational activities.

The advantages of inpatient treatment are constant supervision, active teaching of prosocial behaviors and necessary life skills, and complete isolation from deviant peer groups. The chief disadvantage of inpatient treatment is the student's complete removal from his or her natural setting, and therefore limited likelihood of successfully applying learned skills to environments outside the treatment setting. Although the student may feel competent within the treatment setting, he or she may be unable to perform newly learned behaviors after the treatment is over, given the social pressures occurring within his or her natural environment (Fisher & Harrison, 2005; Stevens & Morral, 2003).

Residential Treatment

On the continuum of treatment options, residential treatment is the most intense option for students with severe substance dependence. Treatment settings include hospitals or other self-contained settings, and are often also referred to as *therapeutic communities*. The defining features of residential treatment are similar to those of inpatient treatment; they include constant supervision, availability of medical detoxification treatment, an isolated setting, a rigidly structured schedule, and intensive counseling designed to increase the student's understanding of the personal and interpersonal consequences of his or her behavior. In comparison to inpatient programs, residential programs are usually longer and can last up to 1 year or more (Fisher & Harrison, 2005).

Upon entry into a residential treatment program, the student becomes part of a rigid social hierarchy where privileges need to be earned and where rewards and punishments are strictly administered based on following or not following program rules. Activities include daily housekeeping and work tasks; counseling sessions; educational activities, such as formal courses of study leading to a general equivalency diploma (GED), conducted by local teaching staff; and extracurricular activities, such as guest speaker presentations on health-related issues or field trips (Stevens & Morral, 2003). Contact with family members is limited and highly regulated. Once program staff reassess the student and determine that he or she has acquired prosocial attitudes and the behavioral skills necessary for a positive lifestyle, the student will be referred to a less intensive treatment setting in preparation for eventual reintegration into his or her natural environment.

Residential treatment is often a last resort for students with the most severe substance dependence. Because of its rigor and long duration, dropout can be high (Fisher & Harrison, 2005). To maximize the likelihood that a student will benefit from the full course of residential treatment, it is therefore important that referrals take into careful consideration the advantages and disadvantages of this treatment option. Advantages of residential treatment include a strictly structured schedule of activities, complete isolation from natural environments and social networks, and intense teaching of prosocial skills. The disadvantages include the disruption of the student's school experience and development within his or her natural environment, due to the length of the treatment. The intensity of the treatment and concomitant risk of not completing it may also limit the benefits the student can derive from residential treatment.

Crisis Plans

If there is an immediate threat to a student's life, the treatment options identified above may not offer necessary assistance in a timely manner. School personnel should develop a crisis plan in collaboration with community agency representatives that assures emergency response and access to medical treatment as needed. In addition to the emergency contacts available in each community, the school personnel and mental health agency personnel may want to collaborate in developing a written plan delineating for responses to life-threatening behaviors, and in educating the students, teachers, administrators, and parents about this plan. For example, if a student suspects that a friend is experiencing an overdose, he or she can call 911 or the poison control center for assistance. Because calls to poison control centers can typically be anonymous, students do not need to fear legal repercussions.

Adolescents involved in substance abuse may often fear legal consequences if they contact emergency personnel to seek help for themselves or others. A crisis plan should allow students to seek immediate help without fear of incrimination. Going through a trusted adult at the school might be one way to get help without directly contacting public authorities. School personnel might be reluctant to make themselves available during nonschool hours to be the first contact and follow-up in emergency situations. However, it is important for all members of the school community to collaborate to identify behaviors and symptoms that require immediate attention, know how to respond, and have recourse for help that they will readily use.

Putting It All Together

Figure 7.1 is a flowchart illustrating the phases, critical features, and important checkpoints of the consultation and referral process. The chart emphasizes the collaborative nature of the process by juxtaposing school and community responsibilities and directing

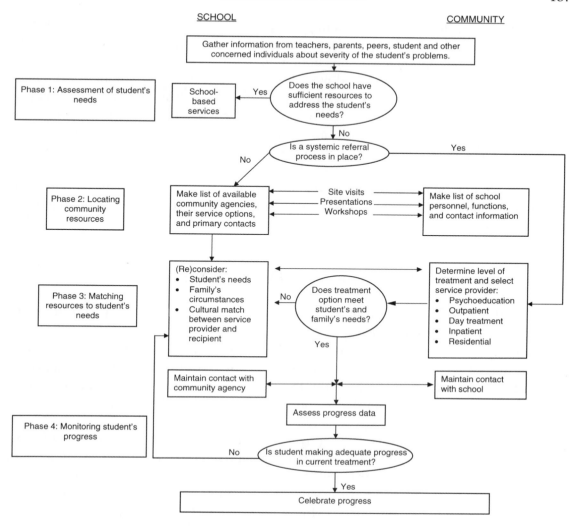

FIGURE 7.1. Coordinating treatment for students with substance abuse and related problems.

the reader back and forth between the two. The process is not linear or unidirectional; some steps occur concurrently, can be omitted, or need to be repeated in certain circumstances. Phase 1 constitutes a needs assessment. Once a school mental health professional encounters a student with a substance abuse problem, he or she assesses whether the school can adequately meet the student's needs. This initial phase of the process includes consultation with members of various school constituencies and an inventory of the school personnel's time, expertise, and resources. If there is a match between the two, the student should receive school-based services. Phase 2 focuses on formal and informal networking to generate a list of community agencies and their services that can be disseminated to students and families, as well as to the entire school community. If the school has a systemic referral process in place and information on community services is readily available, Phase 2 becomes unnecessary. Phase 3 requires school personnel to locate the treatment option along the continuum of services that is most appropriate for the student's substance problem and most likely to succeed. Considerations of the family's individual circumstances and cultural background, as well as confidentiality and privacy for the student and his or her family, should inform this phase of the process. After the student has been referred to a community agency for treatment, it is important that the school and service provider remain in close contact by continually assessing the student's progress (Phase 4). Lack of progress should be promptly addressed by reconsidering the treatment's adequacy for the student's problem or the match between treatment provider and recipient. Adequate progress should be duly noted and appropriately celebrated.

CONSIDERING FINANCIAL RESPONSIBILITIES

Although the consultation and referral process should always be driven by the student's needs and family's circumstances, school personnel also need to be aware of and negotiate financial responsibilities carefully. In general, schools are responsible only for providing educational services. Services that are not directly linked to educational benefits are generally the parents' financial responsibility. Thus a crucial step in determining who is to pay for mental health and substance abuse services is to decide whether those services are necessary for the student's academic progress.

A first step in making this decision is to find out whether the student is eligible for special education and related services and has an *individualized education plan* (IEP). An IEP specifies the services necessary for the student to meet his or her unique educational needs. Services necessary to allow the student to benefit educationally and achieve his or her annual goals must be provided by the school under IDEA. If a student's substance abuse problem is deemed to be due to a documented disability and to prevent the student from making progress toward educational goals, the IEP team might consider substance abuse treatment a "related service" necessary and appropriate for educational benefit.

Substance abuse may occur in conjunction with other medical conditions or disabilities that might make associated treatments part of a free appropriate public education (FAPE), to which all students identified with a disability are entitled under IDEA. An informative and comprehensive website (*www.wrightslaw.com*) offers information on IDEA, FAPE, provision of special education services, and schools' and parents' rights and responsibilities.

The most recent reauthorization of IDEA (2004) presents a complex constellation of circumstances when mental health and substance abuse treatment services might be considered part of special education services. Part C of the Act makes provisions for services for infants and toddlers "affected by illegal substance abuse or withdrawal symptoms resulting from prenatal drug exposure" (Apling & Jones, 2005, p. 41). Responses to complex substance-abuse-related behaviors by middle and high school students are less clearly addressed by the law. The fact that there seems to be a high correlation between emotional and behavioral disorders and substance abuse (McCombs & Moore, 2002) suggests that students with documented diagnoses of these disorders who engage in substance abuse as a direct result of the disorders may be entitled to special services. Whether those services include drug treatment and counseling is unclear. Diagnostic criteria, legal definitions, and source of referral must be carefully considered on a case-by-case basis to sort out financial responsibilities.

If, however, a student is not eligible to receive special education and related services, schools may not be obligated to provide access to services that are not directly related to the student's educational progress. Under these circumstances, financial responsibilities are difficult to sort out and generally are considered the parents' responsibility.

If the school participates in funded drug prevention programs—for example, the Drug Abuse Resistance Education (D.A.R.E.) program—these programs may provide students access to substance abuse services through the school. If a student's substance abuse and related problems are severe, and he or she is at risk of or actually engages in criminal activities, the school might consult with the local or state justice systems to provide and finance appropriate treatment options.

Given these legal complexities, school personnel may be reluctant to refer a student to a treatment for whose cost the school might be held responsible. Although this reluctance is understandable, it should not be the primary consideration in selecting a treatment. The school mental health professional should clearly communicate with the parents regarding treatment costs and financial responsibilities, and should actively work with community agencies to locate appropriate and financially viable treatment options.

BUILDING AND MAINTAINING A SYSTEMIC REFERRAL PROCESS

Although each treatment plan must be individualized, a systemic referral process facilitates proactive approaches to substance abuse, prompts treatment selection once a specific need has been identified, and provides immediate attention to individual students' needs. A systemic approach to substance abuse prevention and treatment requires coordinated collaboration among school, home, and community. The school mental health professional can be the primary liaison among these settings and the "point person" for questions and concerns.

Stable and durable collaborations across multiple sites with potentially different conceptual frameworks and service delivery models should be team-based, mutually educational, and responsive to existing policies (Johnson & Johnson, 2003; Macklem & Kalinski, 2000). These critical features are relevant for building and maintaining a cohesive and responsive consultation and referral system that benefits all members of the school community.

Team-Based Approach

A sustainable consultation and referral system must be collaborative. A team-based approach assures participation from all constituencies of the school community, but also builds continuity in case of personnel changes in the school (Johnson & Johnson, 2003; Sugai & Horner, 2006). The membership of a school-based team will vary, but should be representative of the entire school community. Members might include general and special education teachers, the school counselor and/or school psychologist, at least one administrator, students, and parents. In addition to responding to individual students' needs, the team should be highly visible in the school through regular educational and preventive interactions with the entire school population. It is important that the team has the strong support of the school administration for political leadership and influence within the community. Student participation is equally critical for an effective team, because it increases student ownership of the consultation and referral process. Parent participants are a crucial link to the home environment as well as to the community, and can offer useful perspectives on students' out-of-school activities and whereabouts.

Mutual Education

Once a school-based team is in place and operates regularly and efficiently, structured interactions with community services can be added to the team's responsibilities. Under the guidance of a school mental health professional and with the support of the other team members and community mental health professionals, regular collaborations with community-based treatment agencies can be established and nurtured. Designated team members should locate primary contacts within each agency; arrange personal contacts with the agency, to strengthen and solidify the relationship between school and agency; and invite agency representatives to visit the school and present their agency's goals, approaches, and treatment options to the team. These activities should be mutually educational. They should inform the agency of the school's population characteristics, policies, service capacity, and history with substance-abuse-related behaviors; they should inform the school team of the agency's structure, service delivery approaches, and available treatment options. It is important to maintain regular contact with a service provider to allow mutual updates of personnel changes, as well as changes in services and needs. Contacts with agency representatives might also provide opportunities to review aggregated outcomes of students receiving school-based or community-based treatment to refine referral criteria.

Responsiveness to Existing Policies

Schools rarely operate independently, but rather are part of district and state administrative systems that regulate policies and procedures. As such, school-based teams, under the direction of a school administrator, need to be responsive to district, state, and federal laws or mandates regulating substance abuse treatment policies and procedures. These

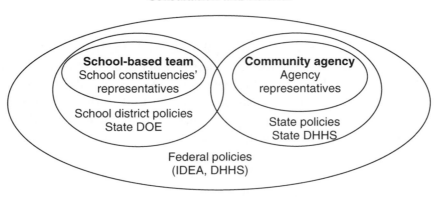

FIGURE 7.2. An integrated systemic approach to consultation and referral. DOE, Department of Education; DHHS, Department of Health and Human Services; IDEA, Individuals with Disabilities Education Act.

laws or mandates may have a major impact on referral procedures, service eligibility criteria, and financial responsibilities. The school team needs to familiarize itself with these larger administrative regulations to facilitate quick, efficient, and appropriate responses to students' needs, as well as to avoid redundancies in service delivery or inaccessibility of needed services due to bureaucratic barriers.

A systemic approach to consultation and referral can be represented as a series of concentric circles incorporating both school and community agencies. Figure 7.2 shows a school-based and a community agency, each embedded in local and state administrative systems relevant to itself, and both embedded in large-scale federal policies. This model should be understood as interactive and dynamic. Policies defining the responsibilities of each component will vary from state to state.

CASE EXAMPLE

This section provides a brief case example of a student whose substance abuse required services that exceeded her school's capacity. The example illustrates some of the steps of the consultation and referral process described above.

Katrina was a 16-year-old student attending 10th grade at Dylan High School in a mid-sized city. Her father was an elementary school teacher who had immigrated from Germany, and her mother worked for a federal government agency. Katrina had excelled in her schoolwork throughout her career as a student, until her teachers and parents noticed a drop in grades beginning in her 9th-grade year. Teachers' attempts to encourage Katrina to complete homework and prepare for tests were always met with enthusiastic reassurances by Katrina that she would do everything it took to improve her performance. However, no improvements were noticeable. Her parents also pleaded with their daughter to spend more time on her schoolwork, but those pleas remained equally ineffective.

In addition to Katrina's declining academic performance, she was beginning to receive an increasing number of office discipline referrals for being under the influence of alcohol on school grounds. Her social studies teacher, who instructed Katrina during the period after the lunch break, smelled alcohol on Katrina's breath several times and referred her to the office for alcohol use. Katrina admitted to the school counselor that she and her friends often purchased beer at a nearby convenience store (where the clerks did not check customers' IDs) during their lunch break and shared it before returning to school. The school counselor met with Katrina several times and, after consultation with her parents, asked her to attend weekly group counseling sessions at school. During these sessions, under the school counselor's supervision and guidance, students learned about the risks of drug use and abuse, health consequences, and potential legal ramifications. Although Katrina attended the counseling sessions regularly, her teachers and parents did not notice any improvements in her behavior; on the contrary, her use of alcohol seemed to increase, and Katrina was late to school several times after staying out late with her friends the night before.

On the advice of Katrina's teachers, the school counselor met again with her parents and recommended that Katrina participate in a local outpatient drug treatment program. Initially, both parents were appalled at the thought that their daughter needed treatment. Katrina's mother was convinced that Katrina was simply going through a phase and would eventually become mature enough to handle alcohol responsibly. After all, her mother maintained, she herself had gone through a similar phase during her high school years, with no lasting detriment to her health and overall welfare. Her father tried to convince the school counselor that U.S. culture is overly concerned about underage alcohol use. In his home country of Germany, it is legal to drink beer and wine at age 16 and hard liquor at age 18, and even these relaxed standards are rarely enforced. Therefore, alcoholic beverages are readily available to German children of all ages and do not possess the "mystique" of the forbidden. Alcohol use among teenagers, Katrina's father insisted, is no problem.

In spite of their initial resistance to the school counselor's recommendation for additional treatment, the counselor was able to convince the parents that treatment was necessary to prevent a further decline in Katrina's academic performance. He presented the parents with a list of community-based agencies offering services that might suit Katrina's needs, and discussed the costs of the most appropriate treatment option with them. The counselor suggested an outpatient program at the Family Development Center, which was located close to Katrina's home and welcomed parental participation in counseling sessions. Through numerous conversations with the program's primary administrator, the counselor knew that the administrator's wife was originally from Germany, and that the administrator was therefore familiar with culturally different attitudes toward alcohol use by minors. Before Katrina began treatment, the counselor, in collaboration with the program's counseling staff, asked Katrina and her parents to consent to the treatment plan by signing a formal consent letter. State law mandated that parent and student consent be on file prior to a student receiving treatment for substance abuse.

Katrina and her parents attended twice-weekly 1-hour counseling sessions at the Family Development Center. Katrina and her parents learned about the long-term risks of alcohol use, strategies to stop the use pattern by substituting other activities, and the importance of developing healthy peer relationships.

After the 10-week program was over, Katrina began to distance herself from her former peer group. Her consumption of alcohol during the lunch breaks became less frequent, because her new friends were not interested in leaving the school grounds during their lunch break, but remained in the cafeteria to play Magic Cards. After about a month, Katrina's teachers were pleased to notice that her grades had stabilized; her office discipline referrals had drastically decreased; and the social studies teacher was no longer concerned about smelling alcohol on Katrina's breath after lunch.

CHAPTER SUMMARY

Given the enormous array of students' needs, schools cannot reasonably be expected to provide adequate substance abuse/mental health services for all students. Linkages with community agencies provide needed services, encourage a sense of shared responsibility, and promote a proactive approach to substance abuse education. School mental health professionals play a pivotal role in establishing and nurturing these linkages through the consultation and referral process. This process usually begins with identifying student needs that exceed the capacity of school-based personnel and gathering critical pieces of information to shape an action plan. Once sufficient information has been collected, available resources must be located and carefully matched to students' individual needs. Individual family characteristics must be considered to shape a treatment plan that is culturally sensitive and that the student is likely to complete.

Non-school-based service options range in intensity from psychoeducation, outpatient treatment, and day treatment to inpatient and residential programs. The advantages and disadvantages of each treatment option need to be carefully considered to maximize treatment benefits. Ongoing contact between the school and the community agency while a student receives treatment facilitates the student's reintegration into the school community after the treatment has been completed. Funding of needed services can be a challenge, particularly for students with multiple diagnoses or identified disabilities. Close consultation with parents or guardians regarding financial responsibilities and eligibility criteria for state-funded services is recommended to make sure that students receive the services they need.

To provide prompt and easy access to community services, schools can build and maintain a sustainable referral system. A team-based approach assures continuity of interagency relationships; mutually educational activities assure access to current information. Administrative policies and procedures governing school and agency service delivery need to be considered to minimize bureaucratic delays and redundancies in service delivery, and to maximize student success.

CHAPTER RESOURCES

The following websites provide useful information for locating local treatment options, building linkages between school and community, and educating students and parents on substance abuse.

Center for Mental Health in Schools, UCLA
smhp.psych.ucla.edu

This website provides information on existing programs, their effectiveness, and research data, as well as networking links.

National Clearinghouse on Alcohol and Drug Information (NCADI)
ncadi.samhsa.gov

This government-hosted website provides information on recent publications, assessment instruments, and research outcomes.

National Institute on Drug Abuse (NIDA)
www.nida.nih.gov

The NIDA website offers information for teachers, parents, and students on drug prevention programs, research data, and recent publications.

Office of Safe and Drug-Free Schools
www.ed.gov/about/offices/list/osdfs/programs.html

This site offers information on federally funded education and prevention programs, as well as links to funding opportunities.

Substance Abuse and Mental Health Services Administration (SAMHSA)
www.samhsa.gov

The main SAMHSA website provides a wealth of information on substance abuse trends, as well as data on specific substances; it also has a link to a treatment locator service allowing visitors to search for services by state and city (see below).

Substance Abuse Treatment Facility Locator
www.findtreatment.samhsa.gov

This SAMHSA-sponsored site includes a comprehensive directory of treatment facilities and programs, searchable by state and city.

Wrightslaw
www.wrightslaw.com

This is a comprehensive site offering information on special education law and advocacy for children with disabilities.

References

Abadinsky, H. (2004). *Drugs: An introduction* (5th ed.). Belmont, CA: Wadsworth/Thomson Learning.

Adelman, H. S., & Taylor, L. (1997). Restructuring education support services and integrating community resources: Beyond the full service school model. *School Psychology Review, 25,* 431–445.

Adelman, H. S., & Taylor, L. (2000). Substance abuse prevention: Toward comprehensive, multifaceted approaches. *Addressing Barriers to Learning, 5*(3), 5–7.

Alberta Alcohol and Drug Abuse Commission. (2003). *Youth risk and protective factors.* Retrieved November 15, 2005, from *http://corp.aadac.com/content/corporate/gambling/YouthRiskProtFactors390U-0.pdf*

Alberto, P. A., & Troutman, A. C. (2003). *Applied behavior analysis for teachers* (6th ed.). Upper Saddle River, NJ: Merrill/Prentice Hall.

Alcoholics Anonymous (AA). (2006). *A brief guide to Alcoholics Anonymous.* Retrieved January 29, 2006, from *www.alcoholics-anonymous.org/en_pdfs/p-42_abriefguidetoaa.pdf*

Allen, J. P., & Wilson, V. B. (Eds.). (2003). *Assessing alcohol problems: A guide for clinicians and researchers* (2nd ed.) (NIH Publication No. 03-3745). Bethesda, MD: National Institute on Alcohol Abuse and Alcoholism.

American Academy of Child and Adolescent Psychiatry (AACAP). (2005). Practice parameter for the assessment and treatment of children and adolescents with substance use disorders. *Journal of the American Academy of Child and Adolescent Psychiatry, 44*(6), 609–621.

American Psychiatric Association. (2000). *Diagnostic and statistical manual of mental disorders* (4th ed., text rev.). Washington, DC: Author.

American Society of Addiction Medicine. (2002). *Patient placement criteria* (2nd ed.). Chevy Chase, MD: Author.

Anthony, J. C., & Petronis, K. R. (1995). Early-onset drug use and risk of later drug problems. *Drug and Alcohol Dependence, 40,* 9–15.

Apling, R., & Jones, N. L. (2005). *Individuals with Disabilities Education Act (IDEA): Analysis of changes made by P.L. 108–446.* Washington, DC: Congressional Research Service.

Arthur, M. W., Hawkins, J. D., Pollard, J. A., Catalano, R. F., & Baglioni, J. A. J. (2002). Measuring risk and protective factors for substance use, delinquency, and other adolescent problem behaviors: The Communities That Care Youth Survey. *Evaluation Review, 26,* 575–601.

Attkisson, C. C., & Greenfield, T. K. (1999). The UCSF Client Satisfaction Scales: I. The Client Satisfaction

Questionnaire–8. In M. E. Maruish (Ed.), *The use of psychological testing for treatment planning and outcome assessment* (pp. 1333–1346). Mahwah, NJ: Erlbaum.

Austin, A. M., Macgowan, M. J., & Wagner, E. F. (2005). Effective family-based interventions for adolescents with substance use problems: A systematic review. *Research on Social Work Practice, 15,* 67–83.

Baer, J. S., & Peterson, P. L. (2002). Motivational interviewing with adolescents and young adults. In W. R. Miller & S. Rollnick, *Motivational interviewing: Preparing people for change* (2nd ed., pp. 320–332). New York: Guilford Press.

Bandura, A. (1977a). Self-efficacy: Toward a unifying theory of behavioral change. *Psychological Review, 84*(2), 191–215.

Bandura, A. (1977b). *Social learning theory.* Englewood Cliffs, NJ: Prentice Hall.

Bandura, A. (1994). Regulative function of perceived self-efficacy. In J. H. Harris (Ed.), *Personnel selection and classification* (pp. 261–271). Hillsdale, NJ: Erlbaum.

Barnes, G. M., & Welte, J. W. (1986). Patterns and predictors of alcohol use among 7–12th grade students in New York State. *Journal of Studies on Alcohol, 47,* 53–62.

Benman, D. S. (1995). Risk factors leading to adolescent substance abuse. *Adolescence, 30,* 201–208.

Botvin, G. J. (1998). Preventing adolescent drug abuse through LifeSkills Training: Theory, methods, and effectiveness. In J. Crane (Ed.), *Social programs that work* (pp. 225–257). New York: Russell Sage Foundation.

Botvin, G. J. (2000). Preventing drug abuse in schools: Social and competence enhancement approaches targeting individual-level etiologic factors. *Addictive Behaviors, 25*(6), 887–897.

Botvin, G. J., Baker, E., Dusenbury, L., Botvin, E. M., & Diaz, T. (1995). Long-term follow-up results of a randomized drug abuse prevention trial in a white middle-class population. *Journal of the American Medical Association, 273,* 1106–1112.

Botvin, G. J., Renick, N., & Baker, E. (1983). The effects of scheduling format and booster sessions on a broad-spectrum psychosocial approach to smoking prevention. *Journal of Behavioral Medicine, 6,* 359–379.

Bronfenbrenner, U. (1979). *The ecology of human development: Experiments by nature and design.* Cambridge, MA: Harvard University Press.

Brook, J. S., Whiteman, M., Gordon, A. S., & Brook, D. W. (1990). The role of older brothers in younger brothers' drug use viewed in the context of parent and peer influences. *Journal of Genetic Psychology, 151,* 59–75.

Brown, S. A. (2001). Facilitating change for adolescent alcohol problems: A multiple options approach. In E. F. Wagner & H. B. Waldron (Eds.), *Innovations in adolescent substance abuse interventions* (pp. 169–187). New York: Pergamon Press.

Burrow-Sanchez, J. (2006). Understanding adolescent substance abuse: Prevalence, risk factors, and clinical implications. *Journal of Counseling and Development, 84,* 283–290.

Burrow-Sanchez, J. J., & Lopez, A. L. (in press). Identifying substance abuse issues in high schools: A national survey of high school counselors. *Journal of Counseling and Development.*

Burrow-Sanchez, J. J., Lopez, A. L., & Slagle, C. P. (in press). Perceived competence in addressing student substance abuse: A national survey of middle school counselors. *Journal of School Health.*

Catalano, R., Hawkins, J. D., Wells, K., & Miller, J. (1990). Evaluation of the effectiveness of adolescent drug abuse treatment, assessment of risks for relapse, and promising approaches for relapse prevention. *International Journal of the Addictions, 25,* 1085–1140.

Center for Substance Abuse Treatment (CSAT). (1999a). *Enhancing motivation for change in substance abuse treatment* (Treatment Improvement Protocol [TIP] Series 35, DHHS Publication No. SMA 99-3285). Washington, DC: U.S. Department of Health and Human Services.

Center for Substance Abuse Treatment (CSAT). (1999b). *Screening and assessing adolescents for substance use disorders* (Treatment Improvement Protocol [TIP] Series 31, DHHS Publication No. SMA 99-3282). Washington, DC: U.S. Department of Health of Health and Human Services.

Center for Substance Abuse Treatment (CSAT). (1999c). *Treatment of adolescents with substance use disorders* (Treatment Improvement Protocol [TIP] Series 32, DHHS Publication No. SMA 99-3283). Washington, DC: U.S. Department of Health of Health and Human Services.

Clayton, R. R. (1992). Transitions in drug use: Risk and protective factors. In M. Glantz & R. Pickens (Eds.), *Vulnerability to drug abuse* (pp. 15–51). Washington, DC: American Psychological Association.

Clayton, R. R., Cattarello, A. M., & Johnstone, B. M. (1996). The effectiveness of Drug Abuse Resistance Education (Project DARE): 5–year follow-up results. *Preventive Medicine, 25*, 307–318.

Clayton, R. R., Leukefeld, C. G., Harrington, N. G., & Cattarello, A. (1996). DARE (Drug Abuse Resistance Education) very popular but not very effective. In C. B. McCoy, L. R. Metsch, & J. A. Inciardi (Eds.), *Intervening with drug-involved youth* (pp. 101–109). Thousand Oaks, CA: Sage.

Cloninger, C. R., Bohman, M., & Sigvardsson, S. (1981). Inheritance of alcohol abuse: Cross-fostering analysis of adopted men. *Archives of General Psychiatry, 38*, 861–868.

Colvin, G., Kame'enui, E. J., & Sugai, G. (1993). Reconceptualizing behavior management and school-wide discipline in general education. *Education and Treatment of Children, 16*(4), 361–381.

Corey, G., Corey, M. S., Callanan, P., & Russell, J. M. (2004). *Group techniques* (3rd ed.). Pacific Grove, CA: Brooks/Cole-Thompson Learning.

Corey, M. S., & Corey, G. (2006). *Groups: Process and practice* (7th ed.). Belmont, CA: Thomson/Brooks/Cole.

Crane, K., & Skinner, B. (2003). Community resource mapping: A strategy for promoting successful transition for youth with disabilities. *Information Brief Assessing Trends and Developments in Secondary Education and Transition, 2*(1), 1–5. Minneapolis, MN: National Center on Secondary Education and Transition. (ERIC Reproduction Service No. ED478263)

Cummings, M. E., & Davies, P. T. (1999). Depressed parents and family functioning: Interpersonal effects and children's functioning and development. In T. Joiner & J. C. Coyne (Eds.), *The interactional nature of depression: Advances in interpersonal approaches* (pp. 299–327). Washington, DC: American Psychological Association.

Deas, D., & Thomas, S. E. (2001). An overview of controlled studies of adolescent substance abuse treatment. *American Journal on Addictions, 10*, 178–189.

Dennis, M., Godley, S. H., Diamond, G., Tims, F. M., Babor, T., Donaldson, J., et al. (2004). The Cannabis Youth Treatment (CYT) study: Main findings from two randomized trials. *Journal of Substance Abuse Treatment, 27*, 197–213.

Dennis, M. L., & McGeary, K. A. (1999, Fall). *Adolescent alcohol and marijuana treatment: Kids need it now* (Tie Communique). Rockville, MD: Center for Substance Abuse Treatment.

Dennis, M. L., Titus, J. C., White, M. K., & Hodgkins, D. (2002). *Global Appraisal of Individual Needs (GAIN) version 5 administration manual*. Retrieved December 28, 2005, from *www.chestnut.org/LI/gain/index.html*

Dent, C. W., Sussman, S., & Stacy, A. W. (2001). Project Towards No Drug Abuse: Generalizability to a general high school sample. *Preventive Medicine, 32*, 514–520.

Diamond, G., Godley, S. H., Liddle, H. A., Sampl, S., Webb, C., Tims, F. M., et al. (2002). Five outpatient treatment models for adolescent marijuana use: A description of the Cannabis Youth Treatment interventions. *Addiction, 97*, 70–83.

Dishion, T. J., & Kavanagh, K. (2003). *Intervening in adolescent problem behavior: A family-centered approach.* New York: Guilford Press.

Dishion, T. J., Kavanagh, K., Schneigher, A., Nelson, S., & Kaufman, N. K. (2002). Preventing early adolescent substance use: A family-centered strategy for the public middle school. *Prevention Science, 3*, 191–201.

Dishion, T. J., McCord, J., & Poulin, F. (1999). When interventions harm: Peer groups and problem behavior. *American Psychologist, 54*, 1–10.

Donnermeyer, J. F., & Wurschmidt, T. N. (1997). Educators' perceptions of the D.A.R.E. program. *Journal of Drug Education, 27*, 259–276.

Dowieko, H. E. (2002). *Concepts of chemical dependency*. Pacific Grove, CA: Brooks/Cole.

Duchnowsky, A., & Kutash, K. (2005). Systems of care. In M. Hersen (Series Ed.), G. Sugai & R. H. Horner (Vol. Eds.), *Encyclopedia of behavior modification and cognitive behavior therapy: Vol. 3. Educational applications* (pp. 1555–1559). Thousand Oaks, CA: Sage.

Dukes, R. L., Stein, J. A., & Ullman, J. B. (1997). Long-term impact of Drug Abuse Resistance Education (D.A.R.E.). *Evaluation Review, 21,* 483–500.

Dukes, R. L., Ullman, J. B., & Stein, J. A. (1996). Three-year follow-up of drug abuse resistance education (D.A.R.E.). *Evaluation Review, 20,* 49–66.

Eber, L., Sugai, G., Smith, C., & Scott, T. M. (2002). Wraparound and positive behavioral interventions and supports in the schools. *Journal of Emotional and Behavioral Disorders, 10*(3), 171–180.

Edwards, R. W., Jumper-Thurman, P., Plested, B. A., Oetting, E. R., & Swanson, L. (2000). Community readiness: Research to practice. *Journal of Community Psychology, 28,* 291–307.

Eggert, L. L., Seyl, C., & Nicholas, L. J. (1990). Effects of a school-based prevention program for potential high school dropouts and drug abusers. *International Journal of the Addictions, 25,* 772–801.

Eggert, L. L., Thompson, E. A., Herting, J. R., & Nicholas, L. J. (1995). Reducing suicide potential among high-risk youth: Tests of a school-based prevention program. *Suicide and Life Threatening Behavior, 25,* 276–296.

Eggert, L. L., Thompson, E. A., Herting, J. R., Nicholas, L. J., & Dicker, B. G. (1994). Preventing adolescent drug abuse and high school dropout through an intensive school-based social network development program. *American Journal of Health Promotion, 8,* 202–214.

Eggert, L. L., Thompson, E. A., Herting, J. R., & Randall, B. P. (2001). Reconnecting youth to prevent drug abuse, school dropout, and suicidal behaviors among high-risk youth. In E. Wagner & H. B. Waldron (Eds.), *Innovations in adolescent substance abuse interventions* (pp. 51–84). New York: Pergamon Press.

Ennett, S. T., Tobler, N. S., Ringwalt, C. L., & Flewelling, R. L. (1994). How effective is drug abuse resistance education?: A meta-analysis of Project DARE outcome evaluations. *American Journal of Public Health, 84,* 1394–1401.

Fisher, G. L., & Harrison, T. C. (2005). *Substance abuse: Information for school counselors, social workers, therapists, and counselors.* Boston: Allyn & Bacon.

Foster, S., Rollefson, M., Doksum, T., Noonan, D., Robinson, G., & Teich, J. (2005). *School mental health services in the United States, 2002–2003* (DHHS Publication No. ADM 05–4068). Rockville, MD: Center for Mental Health Services, Substance Abuse and Mental Health Services Administration.

Fowler, R. E., & Tisdale, P. C. (1992). Special education students as a high-risk group for substance abuse: Teachers' perceptions. *The School Counselor, 40,* 103–108.

Geller, B. (1998). Double-blind and placebo-controlled study of lithium for adolescent bipolar disorders with secondary substance dependency. *Journal of the American Academy of Child and Adolescent Psychiatry, 37*(2), 171–178.

Godley, S. H., Godley, M. D., & Dennis, M. L. (2001). The Assertive Aftercare Protocol for adolescent substance abusers. In E. F. Wagner & H. B. Waldron (Eds.), *Innovations in adolescent substance abuse interventions* (pp. 313–331). New York: Pergamon Press.

Gonet, M. M. (1994). *Counseling the adolescent substance abuser: School-based intervention and prevention.* Thousand Oaks, CA: Sage.

Gorsuch, R. L., & Butler, M. C. (1976). Initial drug abuse: A review of predisposing social psychological factors. *Psychological Bulletin, 83,* 120–137.

Greenbaum, P. E., Foster-Johnson, L., & Petrila, A. (1996). Co-occurring addictive and mental disorders among adolescents: Prevalence research and future directions. *American Journal of Orthopsychiatry, 66,* 52–60.

Greenberg, K. R. (2003). *Group counseling in K–12 schools: A handbook for school counselors.* Boston: Allyn & Bacon.

Hamilton, N. L., Brantley, L. B., Tims, F. M., Angelovich, N., & McDougall, B. (2001). *Family support network for adolescent cannabis users* (DHHS Publication No. [SMA] 01-3488, Cannabis Youth Treatment [CYT] Series, Vol. 3). Rockville, MD: Center for Substance Abuse Treatment, Substance Abuse and Mental Health Services Administration.

Hanson, G., & Venturelli, P. (2001). *Drugs and society* (6th ed.). Sudbury, MA: Jones & Bartlett.

Harrell, A., & Wirtz, P. M. (1989). Screening for adolescent problem drinking: Validation of a multidimensional instrument for case identification. *Psychological Assessment, 1,* 61–63.

Hawkins, J. D., Catalano, R. F., & Miller, J. Y. (1992). Risk and protective factors for alcohol and other drug problems in adolescence and early adulthood: Implications for substance abuse prevention. *Psychological Bulletin, 112*(1), 64–105.

Heath, A. C., & Martin, N. (1988). Teenage alcohol use in the Australian Twin Register: Genetic and social determinants of starting to drink. *Alcoholism, Clinical and Experimental Research, 12*, 735–741.

Hoffmann, D., Brunneman, K. D., Gori, G. B., & Wynder, E. L. (1975). On the carcinogenicity of marijuana smoke. In V. C. Runeckles (Ed.), *Recent advances in photochemistry*. New York: Plenum Press.

Ivey, A. E., & Ivey, M. B. (2003). *Intentional interviewing and counseling: Facilitating client development in a multicultural society* (5th ed.). Pacific Grove, CA: Wadsworth.

Jaffe, A., Brown, J., Komer, P., & Witte, G. (1988). *Relapse prevention for the treatment of problem drinking: A manual for therapists and patients*. Unpublished manuscript, Yale University School of Medicine and University of Connecticut Health Center.

Jellinek, E. M. (1952). Phases of alcohol addiction. *Quarterly Journal of Studies on Alcohol, 13*, 673–684.

Jellinek, E. M. (1960). *The disease concept of alcoholism*. New Haven, CT: Hillhouse Press.

Johnson, G. M., Schoutz, F. C., & Locke, T. P. (1984). Relationships between adolescent drug use and parental drug behaviors. *Adolescence, 19*, 295–299.

Johnson, S., & Johnson, C. (2003). Results-based guidance: A systems approach to student support programs. *Professional School Counseling, 6*(3), 180–184.

Johnston, L. D., O'Malley, P. M., Bachman, J. G., & Schulenberg, J. E. (2004). *Demographic subgroup trends for various licit and illicit drugs, 1975–2003* (Monitoring the Future Occasional Paper No. 60). Ann Arbor, MI: Institute for Social Research.

Johnston, L. D., O'Malley, P. M., Bachman, J. G., & Schulenberg, J. E. (2005). *Monitoring the Future national results on adolescent drug use: Overview of key findings 2004* (NIH Publication No. 05-5726). Bethesda, MD: National Institute on Drug Abuse.

Kadden, R., Carroll, K., Donovan, D., Cooney, N., Monti, P., Abrams, D., et al. (1995). *Cognitive-behavioral coping skills therapy manual: A clinical research guide for therapists treating individuals with alcohol abuse and dependence* (Project MATCH, Vol. 3, DHHS Publication No. 94-3724). Rockville, MD: U.S. Department of Health and Human Services.

Kandel, D. B., & Andrews, K. (1987). Processes of adolescent socialization by parents and peers. *International Journal of the Addictions, 22*, 319–342.

Karacostas, D. D., & Fisher, G. L. (1993). Chemical dependency in students with and without learning disabilities. *Journal of Learning Disabilities, 26*, 491–495.

Kazdin, A. E. (2005). *Parent management training: Treatment for oppositional, aggressive, and antisocial behavior in children and adolescents*. New York: Oxford University Press.

Kendler, K. S. (2001). Twin studies of psychiatric illness: An update. *Archives of General Psychiatry, 58*, 1005–1014.

Knudson, M., Kamara, S., & Louden, J. (1992). *The referral process of school intervention programs in Washington State to alcohol and drug assessment centers: A case study of four high schools*. Olympia: Washington State Department of Social and Health Services Planning, Research and Development, and Data Analysis.

Koch, K. A. (1994). The D.A.R.E. (Drug Abuse Resistance Education) program. In J. A. Lewis (Ed.), *Addictions: Concepts and strategies for treatment* (pp. 359–364). Gaithersburg, MD: Aspen.

Komro, K. A., Perry, C. L., Veblen-Mortenson, S., Stigler, M. H., Bosma, L. M., & Munson, K. A. (2004). Violence-related outcomes of the D.A.R.E. Plus project. *Health Education and Behavior, 31*, 335–354.

Lambie, G. W. (2004). Motivational enhancement therapy: A tool for professional school counselors working with adolescents. *Professional School Counseling, 7*(4), 268–276.

Lambie, G. W., & Rokutani, L. (2002). A systems approach to substance abuse identification and intervention for school counselors. *Professional School Counseling, 5*(5), 353–359.

Levy, D., & Sheflin, N. (1985). The demand for alcoholic beverages: An aggregate time-series analysis. *Journal of Public Policy and Marketing, 4*, 47–54.

Lewis, T. J., & Sugai, G. (1999). Effective behavior support: A systems approach to proactive school-wide management. *Effective School Practices, 17*(4), 47–53.

Liddle, H. A. (2004). Family-based therapies for adolescent alcohol and drug use: Research contributions and future research needs. *Addiction, 99,* 76–92.

LifeSkills Training (LST). (2006). LifeSkills Training website. Retrieved April 14, 2006, from *www. lifeskillstraining.com/index.cfm*

Lynam, D. R., Milich, R., Zimmerman, R., Novak, S. P., Logan, T. K., & Martin, C. (1999). Project DARE: No effects at 10–year follow-up. *Journal of Consulting and Clinical Psychology, 67,* 590–593.

Maag, J. W., Irvin, D. M., Reid, R., & Vasa, S. F. (1994). Prevalence and predictors of substance use: A comparison between adolescents with and without learning disabilities. *Journal of Learning Disabilities, 27,* 223–234.

Macklem, G., & Kalinski, R. (2000). *School consultations: Providing both prevention and intervention services to children and school staff.* Paper presented at the annual meeting of the National Association of School Psychologists, New Orleans, LA.

Maddahian, E., Newcomb, M. D., & Bentler, P. M. (1988). Adolescent drug use and intention to use drugs: Concurrent and longitudinal analyses of four ethnic groups. *Addictive Behaviors, 13,* 191–195.

Marsiglia, F. F., Miles, B. W., Dustman, P., & Sills, S. (2002). Ties that protect: An ecological perspective on Latino/a urban pre-adolescent drug use. *Social Work with Multicultural Youth, 11,* 191–219.

Mayer, G. R. (1995). Preventing antisocial behavior in the schools. *Journal of Applied Behavior Analysis, 28,* 467–478.

Mayer, J., & Filstead, W. J. (1979). The Adolescent Alcohol Involvement Scale: An instrument for measuring adolescent use and misuse of alcohol. *Journal of Studies on Alcohol, 40,* 291–300.

McCombs, K., & Moore, D. (2002). *Substance abuse prevention and intervention for students with disabilities: A call to educators.* Arlington, VA: ERIC Clearinghouse on Disabilities and Gifted Education. (ERIC Document Reproduction Service No. ED469441)

Mensch, B. S., & Kandel, D. B. (1988). Dropping out of high school and drug involvement. *Sociology of Education, 61*(2), 95–113.

Merikangas, K. R., Dierker, L. C., & Szatmari, P. (1998). Psychopathology among offspring of parents with substance use and/or anxiety disorders: A high risk study. *Journal of Child Psychology and Psychiatry, 39,* 711–720.

Miller, W. R., & Rollnick, S. (1991). *Motivational interviewing: Preparing people to change addictive behavior.* New York: Guilford Press.

Miller, W. R., & Rollnick, S. (2002). *Motivational interviewing: Preparing people for change* (2nd ed.). New York: Guilford Press.

Miller, W. R., Zweben, A., DiClemente, C. C., & Rychtarik, R. G. (1994). *Motivational enhancement therapy manual: A clinical research guide for therapists treating individuals with alcohol abuse and dependence* (Project MATCH, Vol. 2 DHHS Publication No. 94-3723). Rockville, MD: U.S. Department of Health and Human Services.

Moberg, D. P. (2000). *The Adolescent Alcohol and Drug Involvement Scale.* Madison, WI: Center for Health Policy and Program Evaluation.

Moberg, D. P., & Hahn, L. (1991). The Adolescent Drug Involvement Scale. *Journal of Adolescent Chemical Dependency, 2,* 75–88.

Monti, P. M., Abrams, D. B., Kadden, R. M., & Cooney, N. L. (1989). *Treating alcohol dependence: A coping skills training guide.* New York: Guilford Press.

Moon, D., Hecht, M., Jackson, K., & Spellers, R. (1999). Ethnic and gender differences and similarities in adolescent drug use and refusals of drug offers. *Substance Use and Misuse, 34*(8), 1059–1083.

Mrazek, P. J., & Haggerty, R. J. (Eds.). (1994). *Reducing risks for mental disorders: Frontiers for prevention intervention research.* Washington, DC: National Academy Press.

Muck, R., Zempolich, K. A., Titus, J. C., Fishman, M., Godley, M. D., & Schwebel, R. (2001). An overview of the effectiveness of adolescent substance abuse treatment models. *Youth and Society, 33*(2), 143–168.

Myers, M. G., Brown, S. A., & Mott, M. A. (1993). Coping as a predictor of adolescent substance abuse treatment outcome. *Journal of Substance Abuse, 5,* 15–29.

National Institute on Alcohol Abuse and Alcoholism (NIDA). (2001). *Alcohol and transportation safety* (Alcohol Alert No. 52). Bethesda, MD: Author.

National Institute on Drug Abuse (NIDA). (2003). *Commonly abused drugs card* (AVD No. 137). Bethesda, MD: Author.

National Institute on Drug Abuse (NIDA). (2004a). *NIDA infofacts: Inhalants.* Bethesda, MD: Author.

National Institute on Drug Abuse (NIDA). (2004b). *NIDA infofacts: Marijuana.* Bethesda, MD: Author.

National Institute on Drug Abuse (NIDA). (2005a). *NIDA infofacts: Club drugs.* Bethesda, MD: Author.

National Institute on Drug Abuse (NIDA). (2005b). *NIDA infofacts: Cocaine.* Bethesda, MD: Author.

National Institute on Drug Abuse (NIDA). (2005c). *NIDA infofacts: Heroin.* Bethesda, MD: Author.

National Institute on Drug Abuse (NIDA). (2005d). *NIDA infofacts: LSD.* Bethesda, MD: Author.

National Institute on Drug Abuse (NIDA). (2005e). *NIDA infofacts: Methamphetamine.* Bethesda, MD: Author.

National Institute on Drug Abuse (NIDA). (2005f). *NIDA infofacts: Prescription pain and other medications.* Bethesda, MD: Author.

National Institute on Drug Abuse (NIDA). (2006). *NIDA infofacts: Rohypnol and GHB.* Bethesda, MD: Author.

Newcomb, M. D. (1995). Identifying high-risk youth: Prevalence and patterns of adolescent drug abuse. In E. Rahdert & D. Czechowicz (Eds.), *Adolescent drug abuse: Clinical assessment and therapeutic interventions* (DHHS Publication No. 95-3908, NIDA Research Monograph No. 156, pp. 7–38). Rockville, MD: U.S. Department of Health and Human Services.

O'Brian, C. P., Anthony, J. C., Carroll, K., Childress, A. R., Dackis, C., & Diamond, G. (2005). Defining substance use disorders. In C. P. O'Brian (Ed.), *Treating and preventing adolescent mental health disorders* (pp. 336–389). New York: Oxford University Press.

Pagliaro, A. M., & Pagliaro, L. A. (1996). *Substance use among children and adolescents.* New York: Wiley.

Pentz, M. A. (1998). *Costs, benefits, and cost-effectiveness of comprehensive drug abuse prevention* (Cost–Benefit/Cost-Effectiveness Research of Drug Abuse Prevention: Implications for Programming and Policy, No. 176). Bethesda, MD: National Institute on Drug Abuse.

Pollock, V. E., Schneider, L. S., Gabrielli, W. F., & Goodwin, D. W. (1987). Sex of parent and offspring in the transmission of alcoholism: A meta-analysis. *Journal of Nervous and Mental Disease, 173,* 668–673.

Prochaska, J., & DiClemente, C. (1984). *The transtheoretical approach: Crossing traditional boundaries of therapy.* Homewood, IL: Dow Jones–Irwin.

Rahdert, E. (Ed.). (1991). *The adolescent assessment/referral system manual* (DHHS Publication No. ADM 91-1735). Rockville, MD: National Institute on Drug Abuse.

Riggs, J. D., & Davies, R. D. (2002). A clinical approach to integrating treatment for adolescent depression and substance use. *Journal of the American Academy of Child and Adolescent Psychiatry, 41,* 1253–1255.

Riggs, P. D. (2003). Treating adolescents for substance abuse and comorbid psychiatric disorders. *NIDA Science and Practice Perspectives, 2*(1), 18–28.

Robertson, E. B., David, S. L., & Rao, S. A. (2003). *Preventing drug use among children and adolescents: A research-based guide for parents, educators, and community leaders* (NIH Publication No. 04-4212A). Bethesda, MD: National Institute on Drug Abuse.

Rones, M., & Hoagwood, K. (2000). School-based mental health services: A research review. *Clinical Child and Family Psychology Review, 3,* 223–241.

Rotgers, F. (2003). Cognitive-behavioral theories of substance abuse. In F. Rotgers, J. Morgenstern, & S. T. Walters (Eds.), *Treating substance abuse: Theory and technique* (2nd ed., pp. 166–189). New York: Guilford Press.

Rutherford, M., & Banta-Green, C. (1998). *Effectiveness standards for the treatment of chemical dependency in juvenile offenders: A review of the literature.* Retrieved December 28, 2005, from http://depts.washington.edu/adai/pubs/tr/9801/TechRpt.pdf

Saffer, H., & Grossman, M. (1987). Beer taxes, the legal drinking age, and youth motor vehicle fatalities. *Journal of Legal Studies, 16,* 351–374.

Sales, A. (2004). *Preventing substance abuse: A guide for school counselors.* Greensboro, NC: Caps Press.

Sampl, S., & Kadden, R. (2000). *Motivational enhancement therapy and cognitive behavioral therapy for adolescent cannabis users* (Cannabis Youth Treatment [CYT] Series, Vol. 1, DHHS Publication No. SMA

01-3486). Rockville, MD: Center for Substance Abuse Treatment, Substance Abuse and Mental Health Services Administration. (Available at *www.chestnut.org/LI/cyt/products/mcb5_cyt_v1.pdf*)

Scott, D. M., Surface, J. L., Friedli, D., & Barlow, T. W. (1999). Effectiveness of student assistance programs in Nebraska schools. *Journal of Drug Education, 29*, 165–174.

Schwartz, R. H., & Wirtz, P. W. (1990). Potential substance abuse: Detection among adolescent patients using the Drug and Alcohol Problem (DAP) Quick Screen, a 30-item questionnaire. *Clinical Pediatrics, 29*, 38–43.

Sexton, T. L., & Alexander, J. F. (2000, December). Functional family therapy. *Office of Juvenile Justice and Delinquency Prevention, Juvenile Justice Bulletin*, pp. 3–7.

Shelder, J., & Block, J. (1990). Adolescent drug use and psychological health: A longitudinal inquiry. *American Psychologist, 45*(5), 612–630.

Sher, K. J. (1991). *Children of alcoholics: A critical appraisal of theory and research.* Chicago: University of Chicago Press.

Sheridan, S. M. (2000). Considerations of multiculturalism and diversity in behavioral consultation with parents and teachers. *School Psychology Review, 29*(3), 344–353.

Shin, H. B. (2005). *School enrollment—social and economic characteristics of students: October 2003.* Washington, DC: U.S. Bureau of the Census.

Skiba, R. J. (2000). *Zero tolerance, zero evidence: An analysis for school disciplinary practice* (Policy Research Report No. SRS2). Bloomington: Indiana Education Policy Center.

Skiba, R. J., & Peterson, R. L. (1999). The dark side of zero tolerance: Can punishment lead to safe schools? *Phi Delta Kappa, 80*, 372–376.

Sobell, M. B., & Sobell, L. C. (1993). *Problem drinkers: Guided self-change treatment.* New York: Guilford Press.

Spoth, R., Guyull, M., & Day, S. (2002). Universal family-focused interventions in alcohol-use disorder prevention: Cost-effectivness and cost–benefit analyses of two interventions. *Journal of Studies on Alcohol, 63*, 219–228.

Sridhar, K. S., Raub, W. A., Jr., Weatherby, N. L., Metsch, L. R., Surratt, H. L., Inciardi, J. A., et al. (1994). Possible role of marijuana smoking as a carcinogen in the development of lung cancer at a young age. *Journal of Psychoactive Drugs, 26*, 285–288.

Steinberg, K. S., Carroll, K., Roffman, R. A., & Kadden, R. M. (1997). *Marijuana treatment project therapist manual.* Unpublished manuscript, University of Connecticut l Health Center.

Stevens, S. J., & Morral, A. R. (Eds.). (2003). *Adolescent substance abuse treatment in the United States: Exemplary models from a national evaluation study.* New York: Haworth Press.

Stinchfield, R. D. (1997). Reliability of adolescent self-report pretreatment alcohol and other drug use. *Substance Use and Misuse, 32*, 63–76.

Stormshak, E. A., Dishion, T. J., Light, J., & Yasui, M. (2005). Implementing family-centered interventions within the public middle school: Linking service delivery to change in student problem behavior. *Journal of Abnormal Child Psychology, 33*, 723–733.

Substance Abuse and Mental Health Services Administration (SAMHSA), Office of Applied Studies. (2003). *Results from the 2002 National Survey on Drug Use and Health: National findings* (NHSDA Series H-22, DHHS Publication No. SMA 03-3836). Rockville, MD: Author.

Substance Abuse and Mental Health Services Administration (SAMHSA), Office of Applied Studies. (2004). *Results from the 2003 National Survey on Drug Use and Health: National findings* (NSDUH Series H-25, DHHS Publication No. SMA 04-3964). Rockville, MD: Author.

Sue, D. W., Carter, R. T., Casas, J. M., Fouad, N. A., Ivey, A. E., & Jensen, M. (1998). *Multicultural counseling competencies: Individual and organizational development* (Vol. 11). Thousand Oaks, CA: Sage.

Sugai, G., & Horner, R. H. (2006). A promising approach for expanding and sustaining school-wide positive behavior support. *School Psychology Review, 35*(2), 245–259.

Sugai, G., Horner, R. H., & Gresham, F. M. (2002). Behaviorally effective school environments. In M. R. Shin, H. M. Walker, & G. Stoner (Eds.), *Interventions for academic and behavior problems II: Preventive and remedial approaches.* Bethesda, MD: National Association of School Psychologists.

Sullivan, P., & Kendler, K. (1999). The genetic epidemiology of smoking. *Nicotine and Tobacco Research, 1,* 51–57.

Sussman, S., Dent, C. W., & Stacy, A. W. (2002). Project Towards No Drug Abuse: A review of the findings and future directions. *American Journal of Health Behavior, 26,* 354–365.

Sussman, S., Dent, C. W., Stacy, A. W., & Craig, S. (1998). One-year outcomes of Project Toward No Drug Abuse. *Preventive Medicine, 27,* 632–642.

Tarter, R. E. (2002). Etiology of adolescent substance abuse: A developmental perspective. *American Journal on Addictions, 11,* 171–191.

Taylor-Greene, S., Brown, D., Nelson, L., Longton, J., Gassman, T., Cohen, J., et al. (1997). School-wide behavioral support: Starting the year off right. *Journal of Behavioral Education, 7,* 99–112.

Tobler, N. S. (1992). *Meta-analysis of adolescent drug prevention programs: Final report.* Rockville, MD: National Institute on Drug Abuse.

Tsuang, M. T., Bar, J. L., Harley, R. M., & Lyons, M. J. (2001). The Harvard twin study of substance use: What have we learned? *Harvard Review of Psychiatry, 9,* 267–279.

Turnbull, R., Turnbull, A., Shank, M., & Smith, S. J. (2004). *Exceptional lives: Special education in today's schools* (4th ed.). Upper Saddle River, NJ: Pearson/Merrill/Prentice Hall.

U.S. Bureau of the Census. (2004). Selected characteristics of people at specified levels of poverty in the past 12 months. Retrieved January 15, 2006, from *http://factfinder.census.gov*

van den Bree, M. B., Johnson, E. O., Neale, M. C., & Pickens, R. W. (1998). Genetic and environmental influences on drug use and abuse/dependence in male and female twins. *Drug and Alcohol Dependence, 52,* 231–241.

Vega, W. A., & Gil, A. G. (1998). *Drug use and ethnicity in early adolescence.* New York: Plenum Press.

Wagner, E. F., Brown, S. A., Monti, P. M., Myers, M. G., & Waldron, H. B. (1999). Innovations in adolescent substance abuse intervention. *Alcoholism: Clinical and Experimental Research, 23,* 236–249.

Waldron, H. B., Brody, J. L., & Slesnick, N. (2001). Integrative behavioral and family therapy for adolescent substance abuse. In P. M. Monti, S. M. Colby, & T. A. O'Leary (Eds.), *Adolescents, alcohol, and substance abuse: Reaching teens through brief interventions* (pp. 216–243). New York: Guilford Press.

Waldron, H. B., & Kaminer, Y. (2004). On the learning curve: The emerging evidence supporting cognitive-behavioral therapies for adolescent substance abuse. *Addiction, 99*(Suppl. 2), 93–105.

Walker, H. M., Horner, R. H., Sugai, G., Bullis, M., Sprague, J. R., & Bricker, D. (1996). Integrated approaches to preventing antisocial behavior patterns among school-age children and youth. *Journal of Emotional and Behavioral Disorders, 4,* 194–209.

Wallace, J. M., Jr., Bachman, J. G., O'Malley, P. M., Schulenberg, J. E., Cooper, S. M., & Johnston, L. D. (2003). Gender and ethnic differences in smoking, drinking and illicit drug use among American 8th, 10th and 12th grade students, 1976–2000. *Addiction, 98,* 225–234.

Wallace, J. M., Jr., & Muroff, J. R. (2002). Preventing substance abuse among african American children and youth: Race differences in risk factor exposure and vulnerability. *Journal of Primary Prevention, 22,* 235–265.

Webb, C., Scudder, M., Kaminer, Y., & Kadden, R. (2002). *The motivational enhancement therapy and cognitive behavioral therapy supplement: 7 sessions of cognitive behavioral therapy for adolescent cannabis users* (Cannabis Youth Treatment [CYT] Series, Vol. 2, DHHS Publication No. ADM 02-3659). Rockville, MD: Center for Substance Abuse Treatment, Substance Abuse and Mental Health Services Administration.

Weber, M. D., Graham, J. W., Hansen, W. B., Flay, B. R., & Johnston, C. A. (1989). Evidence for two paths of alcohol use onset in adolescents. *Addictive Behaviors, 14,* 399–408.

Weinburg, N. Z. (2001). Risk factors for adolescent substance abuse. *Journal of Learning Disabilities, 34,* 343–351.

Westra, M. (1996). *Active communication.* Pacific Grove, CA: Brooks/Cole.

White, H. R., & Labouvie, E. W. (1989). Towards the assessment of adolescent problem drinking. *Journal of Studies on Alcohol, 50,* 30–37.

Williams, R. J., & Chang, S. Y. (2000). A comprehensive and comparative review of adolescent substance abuse treatment outcome. *Clinical Psychology: Science and Practice, 7,* 138–166.

Windle, M. (1999). *Alcohol use among adolescents* (Vol. 42). Thousand Oaks, CA: Sage.

Winters, K. C. (1992). Development of an adolescent alcohol and other drug abuse screening scale: Personal Experience Screening Questionnaire. *Addictive Behaviors, 17,* 479–490.

Winters, K. C. (2001). Assessing adolescent substance use problems and other areas of functioning: State of the art. In P. M. Monti, S. M. Colby, & T. A. O'Leary (Eds.), *Adolescents, alcohol, and substance abuse: Reaching teens through brief interventions* (pp. 80–108). New York: Guilford Press.

Winters, K. C., Stinchfield, R. D., Henly, G. A., & Schwartz, R. H. (1992). Validity of adolescent self-report of alcohol and other drug involvement. *International Journal of the Addictions, 25,* 1379–1395.

Wood, D. (2003). *Patterns of substance abuse among school-age children: Clinical paper.* Retrieved August 28, 2005, from *www.mental-health-matters.com*

Yagamuchi, K., & Kandel, D. B. (1984). Patterns of drug use from adolescence to young adulthood: 3. Patterns of progression. *American Journal of Public Health, 74,* 673–681.

Index

Page numbers followed by *f* indicate figure, *t* indicate table

AA (Alcoholics Anonymous), 26, 132–133
AADIS (Adolescent Alcohol and Drug Involvement Scale), 63–64, 64*t*
AAIS (Adolescent Alcohol Involvement Scale), 64*t*
Academic placement, 109, 149–150*f*
ACC (Assertive Continuing Care), 110
Accountability, administration, 166
Actiq, 46–48*t*
Active listening, 139
Activities, group interventions and, 148, 149–150*f*
ADHD, 5
ADI (Adolescent Drinking Index), 64*t*
ADIS (Adolescent Drug Involvement Scale), 64*t*
Administration
  accountability and, 166
  implementation planning and, 85–91
  of prevention programs, 73
  school policies and. *See* School policy
  support from, 157
Adolescent Alcohol and Drug Involvement Scale (AADIS), 63–64, 64*t*
Adolescent Alcohol Involvement Scale (AAIS), 64*t*
Adolescent Drinking Index (ADI), 64*t*
Adolescent Drug Involvement Scale (ADIS), 64*t*
Adolescent Transitions Program (ATP), 79–81
Aftercare planning, 106, 110, 131–132
Agency capacity, 178
Agreement, student, 56
Alcohol
  disease model and, 26–27
  lifetime prevalence rates and, 7*f*, 8*f*, 9*f*, 11*f*, 14*f*, 15*f*
  substance abuse and, 45–49, 46–48*t*
  See also Substance use
Alcoholics Anonymous (AA), 26, 132–133
Amphetamines, 46–48*t*, 50
Amytal, 46–48*t*
Antidepressants, 99

Anxiety, 124
Assent, student, 56
Assertive Aftercare Protocol, 110
Assertive Continuing Care (ACC), 110
Assessment
  defining, 57–58
  determining need for, 61*f*
  functional, 102–103
  needs identification and, 64–65
  pretreatment, 111*t*, 113–114
  See also Intervention; Screening
Ativan, 46–48*t*
ATP (Adolescent Transitions Program), 79–81
Attendance, group interventions and, 153–154
Attention-deficit/hyperactivity disorder (ADHD)
  co-occurrence with substance use and, 5, 63
  as individual factor, 33
  individual interventions and, 97, 123–124
  residential settings and, 99
  Ritalin and, 51
Atypical antidepressants, 99
Authorization for Release of Confidential Information, 19*f*
Availability, school professional's role and, 167–168
Awareness, problem, 88, 90*f*

Barbituates, 5, 46–48*t*, 49. *See also* Substance use
Basic counseling skills (BCS), 139–142
BCS (basic counseling skills), 139–142
Behavior contracts, 103
Behavioral theory, substance abuse and, 29
Behavioral therapy, 102–103
Benzodiazepines, 46–48*t*, 49
Biologically based theories of substance abuse, 26–28
Biphetamine, 46–48*t*
Bipolar disorder, 5
Body language, 139
Brain chemistry, substance abuse and, 27–28

Cannabis, 46–48t, 53–54. *See also* Marijuana
Cannabis Youth Treatment (CYT) project, 112–114
Case examples, 21–23, 29–31, 35–36, 39–42, 41t, 65–67,
    91–93, 124–126, 144, 155–160, 180–182, 191–193
Case manager, role of, 106
CBT. *See* Cognitive-behavioral therapy (CBT)
Central nervous system (CNS)
    depressants and, 45, 50
    narcotics and, 52
Change
    maintenance of, 121–122
    motivation for, 114–121, 117f, 180–182
Cigarettes, 7f, 9f, 11f, 14f, 15f, 46–48t. *See also* Substance
    use
Cigars, 46–48t
Closed-ended questions, 140
Club drugs, 46–48t, 52–53
CNS. *See* Central nervous system (CNS)
Cocaine
    lifetime prevalence rates and, 7f, 8f, 9f, 11f, 14f, 15f
    as a stimulant, 50–51
    substance abuse and, 46–48t
    See also Substance use
Codeine, 46–48t, 51–52
Cognitive-behavioral theories, substance abuse and, 29
Cognitive-behavioral therapy (CBT), 102–103, 105, 111t,
    124
Co-leadership, group interventions and, 153
Collaboration. *See* Consultation
Commitment, individual interventions and, 111t
Communication
    between agencies, 173
    skills for, 115, 149–150f
    Student Screening Decision Sheet (SSDS) and, 61f
Communities That Care Youth Survey, 92
Community factors
    consultation/referral to community-based services. *See*
      Consultation
    needs identification and, 166–170, 187f
    prevention and, 72, 72–73
    risk/protective factors and, 34t, 38–39, 41t
    school collaboration and, 91
    self-help groups and, 132–133
Conduct disorder, 5, 99
Confidentiality
    case examples and, 158–160
    collaboration and, 172–173
    consent and, 56, 176
    Family Educational Rights and Privacy Act (FERPA)
      and, 16–17
    42 CFR, 17–20, 56, 172–173, 174, 176
    group interventions and, 154–156
    sample release of information form and, 19f
Confirmation, of prevention programs, 89, 90f
Confrontation, 142–143
Consent, 56, 176. *See also* Confidentiality
Consultation
    case examples and, 191–193
    coordination of treatment and, 186–188, 187f
    information gathering and, 170–176
    key features of, 164–166

    matching services and, 179–186
    needs identification and, 166–170
    overview of, 163–164
    resource location and, 177–179
    systemic process of, 189–191, 191f
Content
    as aspect of prevention programs, 73–74
    Drug Abuse Resistance Education Program (D.A.R.E.)
      and, 84
    group interventions and, 148, 149–150f
    indicated prevention programs and, 77, 78
    three-tiered prevention programs and, 80
    universal prevention programs and, 75
Co-occurrence of substance use with other disorders, 5,
    106, 123–124. *See also specific disorders*
Coping skills, 29–30, 111t
Counseling skills, 139–142
Crack, 51. *See also* Cocaine
Crisis plans, 186
Cultural considerations
    case examples and, 158–160
    consultation/referral and, 165, 174–176
    group interventions and, 145–147
    individual interventions and, 124
    lifetime prevalence rates and, 12f, 13f, 14f, 15f
    prevention and, 72
    rapport building and, 139–140
    rates of substance use and, 12–14
CYT project, 112–114

DAP (Drug and Alcohol Problem Quick Screen), 64t
D.A.R.E., 81–85, 189
Data collection, 87–88, 173–174
Data-driven approach to intervention, 165–166
Date rape drug. *See* Rohypnol
Day treatment, 100, 108f, 181t, 183–184, 187f
Decisional balance, 114, 116f, 120f
Decision-making skills, group interventions and, 149–150f
Delivery
    as aspect of prevention programs, 73–74
    Drug Abuse Resistance Education Program (D.A.R.E.)
      and, 84
    indicated prevention programs and, 77, 78
    three-tiered prevention programs and, 80
    universal prevention programs and, 75
Delta-9-tetrahydrocannabinol (THC), 53
Denial, of problem, 88–89, 90f
Dependence. *See* Substance dependence
Depressants, 45–50, 46–48t
Depression
    co-occurrence with substance use and, 5
    as individual factor, 36
    individual interventions and, 97
    pharmacotherapy and, 99
    residential settings and, 99
    risk/protective factors and, 33
Desoxyn, 46–48t
Developmental process of groups, 133–138, 134f
Dexedrine, 46–48t
Diagnostic and Statistical Manual of Mental Disorders, 4
Disabilities, substance use and, 14–15

Disease model of substance abuse, 26–27
Disorder, defined, 3–4
Documentation. *See* Data collection
Dopamine, substance abuse and, 27
Dropouts, substance use and, 10
Drug Abuse Resistance Education Program (D.A.R.E.), 81–
    85, 189
Drug and Alcohol Problem Quick Screen (DAP), 64*t*
Drug use. *See* Substance use
DSM-IV-TR, 4
Duragesic, 46–48*t*

Ecological model of development, 31–32, 32*f*
Economic considerations, 188–189. *See also* Socioeconomic
    status
Ecstasy, 7*f*, 8*f*, 9*f*, 46–48*t*, 52–53. *See also* Substance use
Education, mutual, 190
Elementary school, prevention programming and, 72
Empathy, 115
Engagement, individual interventions and, 106
Environmental considerations, 29–31, 31–32. *See also*
    Family factors; Peer factors; School factors
Ethnic considerations
    case examples and, 158–160
    consultation/referral and, 165, 174–176
    group interventions and, 145–147
    individual interventions and, 124
    lifetime prevalence rates and, 12*f*, 13*f*, 14*f*, 15*f*
    prevention and, 72
    rapport building and, 139–140
    rates of substance use and, 12–14
Evaluation
    Drug Abuse Resistance Education Program (D.A.R.E.)
        and, 81–85
    group interventions and, 148–151
    of prevention programs, 73–81
    self, 180–182
Expansion, of prevention programs, 89, 90*f*
Expectations, self-efficacy and, 30–31
Experimental substance use, 2–3, 6–8, 7*f*, 35, 181*t*

Faith-based groups, 132–133
Family Educational Rights and Privacy Act (FERPA), 16–17
Family factors
    family involvement and, 122–123
    family-based treatment and, 103
    group interventions and, 154–156
    individual interventions and, 106
    integrated behavioral and family therapy and, 105
    problems in family and, 3
    residential settings and, 99–100
    risk/protective factors and, 34*t*, 35–36, 41*t*
FAPE (free appropriate public education), 188
Federal laws
    Family Educational Rights and Privacy Act (FERPA),
        16–17
    42 CFR, 17–20, 56, 172–173, 174, 176
    Gun-Free Schools Act (GFSA), 20
    systemic process of consultation/referral and, 189–191, 191*f*
Fentanyl, 46–48*t*
FERPA (Family Educational Rights and Privacy Act), 16–17

Financial considerations, 188–189. *See also* Socioeconomic status
Flunitrazepam, 46–48*t*, 49
Follow-up, 61*f*, 65. *See also* Aftercare planning; Evaluation
42 CFR, 17–20, 56, 172–173, 174, 176
Free appropriate public education (FAPE), 188
Functional assessment, 102–103, 119*f*

GAIN (Global Appraisal of Individual Needs), 113–114, 125
Gamma-hydroxybutyrate (GHB), 46–48*t*, 49–50, 52–53
Gases, 46–48*t*, 55
Gender considerations, 10–11, 11*f*
Genetic factors, substance abuse and, 28
GFSA (Gun-Free Schools Act), 20
GHB, 46–48*t*, 49–50, 52–53
Global Appraisal of Individual Needs (GAIN), 113–114, 125
Goal-setting
    group interventions and, 148, 149–150*f*, 156–157
    individual interventions and, 111*t*
    Personal Goal Worksheet, 118*f*
    psychoeducation and, 180–182
Group interventions
    case examples and, 158–160
    developmental process of groups and, 133–138, 134*f*
    leadership skills and, 138–147
    practical considerations for, 147–158
    types of, 130–133
Gun-Free Schools Act (GFSA), 20

Halcion, 46–48*t*
Hallucinogens
    lifetime prevalence rates and, 7*f*, 8*f*, 9*f*, 11*f*, 14*f*, 15*f*
    as substances, 3
    See also Substance use
Harm reduction, 98
Hashish, 46–48*t*, 53–54. *See also* Marijuana
Heroin, 11*f*, 14*f*, 15*f*, 46–48*t*, 51–52. *See also* Substance use
High school, prevention programming and, 72
Hydrochlorine, 46–48*t*
Hydrocodone bitartrate with acetaminophen, 46–48*t*

IDEA (Individuals with Disabilities Education Act), 167–
    168, 188–189
IEPs. *See* Individualized education plans (IEPs)
Implementation
    individual interventions and, 106–107
    of prevention programs, 85–91, 90*f*
Indicated prevention programs, 70–71, 70*f*, 75–77, 77–79.
    See also Three-tiered prevention programs
Individual factors, risk/protective factors and, 33, 34*t*, 41*t*
Individual interventions
    adaptation of CYT project and, 113–122
    basis for sample program, 112–113
    case examples and, 124–126
    components of, 106
    current treatment and, 98–104
    effectiveness of current interventions and, 104–106
    implementation of, 106–107
    overview of, 96–97
    school professional's role and, 107–110, 108*f*
    Suggested Structure for Intervention Based upon MET
        and CBT, 111*t*

Individualized education plans (IEPs), 107, 188
Individuals with Disabilities Education Act (IDEA), 167–168, 188–189
Information dissemination, 179
Information gathering, consultation/referral and, 170–176, 187f
Inhalants
    lifetime prevalence rates and, 7f, 8f, 9f, 11f, 14f, 15f
    substance abuse and, 46–48t, 54–55
    See also Substance use
Initial stage of a group, 134–136, 134f
Initiation, of prevention programs, 89, 90f
Inpatient treatment settings, 99–100, 108f, 181t, 184–185, 187f
Instruments, screening, 63–64, 64t
Integrated behavioral and family therapy, 105, 108f
Intervention
    assessment and, 57
    collaboration and, 165
    consultation/referral and. See Consultation
    group. See Group interventions
    individual. See Individual interventions
    types of, 1
Interviewing
    group interventions and, 152–153
    screening and, 62–63

Junior high school, prevention programming and, 72

Ketamine, 52–53

Large group guidance, 131–132
Leadership skills, 138–147, 153
Learned behaviors, 102–103
Learning disorders, 39–42. See also Attention-deficit/
    hyperactivity disorder (ADHD)
Legal considerations
    case examples and, 191–193
    Family Educational Rights and Privacy Act (FERPA), 16–17
    42 CFR, 17–20, 56, 172–173, 174, 176
    group interventions and, 154
    Gun-Free Schools Act (GFSA), 20
    systemic process of consultation/referral and, 189–191, 191f
Librium, 46–48t
LifeSkills Training (LST), 74–75, 93
Lifetime prevalence rates, 7f, 8f, 9f, 11f, 14f, 15f
Listening skills, 115, 139
Logistics, group, 148, 149–150f, 151–154
LSD, 3, 46–48t, 52–53. See also Substance use
LST. See LifeSkills Training (LST)
Lysergic acid diethylamide (LSD), 3, 46–48t, 52–53. See also Substance use

Marijuana
    case examples and, 22
    lifetime prevalence rates and, 7f, 8f, 9f, 11f, 14f, 15f
    substance abuse and, 53–54
    as substance of abuse, 46–48t
    as substances, 3
    See also Substance use

MDMA, 7f, 8f, 9f, 46–48t, 52–53. See also Substance use
Measures, screening, 63–64, 64t
Medial forebrain bundle, substance abuse and, 27
Medication. See also Pharmacotherapy
Medication, residential settings and, 99
Mental health professionals' role
    group interventions and, 132
    individual interventions and, 106–107
    screening and, 55–60
MET (motivational enhancement therapy), 103–104, 105, 111t
Methamphetamine
    co-occurrence with substance use and, 5
    lifetime prevalence rates and, 7f, 8f, 9f
    substance abuse and, 46–48t
    as substances, 3
    See also Substance use
Methaqualone, 46–48t, 50
Methylenedioxyme thamphetamine, 7f, 8f, 9f, 46–48t, 52–53. See also Substance use
Methylphenidate, 3, 46–48t, 51
Middle school, prevention programming and, 72
Minnesota model, 101–102
Modeling, 30, 142
Monitoring, 61f, 187f
Morphine, 46–48t, 51–52
Motivation, 106, 111t, 114–121, 180–182
Motivational enhancement therapy (MET), 103–104, 105, 111t
Mushrooms, 52–53
Mutual education, 190

Narcotics, 3, 46–48t, 51–52. See also Substance use
Needs analysis
    assessment and, 64–65
    community-based services and, 166–170
    of student, 173–174, 187f
Neighborhoods. See Community factors
Nembutal, 46–48t
Neurotransmitters, substance abuse and, 27
Nicotine, 46–48t. See also Cigarettes
Nitrites, 46–48t, 55
Nonverbal communication, 139

Open-ended questions, 140
Opiates. See Narcotics
Opioids. See Narcotics
Opium, 46–48t
Outcomes
    consultation/referral and, 166, 168–169
    group interventions and, 148–151
Outpatient treatment settings, 100, 108f, 181t, 182–183, 187f
Oxycodone, 46–48t
OxyContin, 3, 46–48t, 52. See also Substance use

Pain medication, 3. See also Substance use
Paraphrasing skills, 140–142
Parent education, 123
Parent management training programs, 103
Parents
    collaboration and, 170–173
    consent of, 56, 176
    requests for help from, 169–170

skills of, 36
  See also Family factors
Parest, 46–48*t*
Partial hospitalization, 100, 108*f*
Paxil, 99
Peer factors
  collaboration and, 170–173
  individual interventions and, 106
  requests for help from, 169–170
  risk/protective factors and, 33–35, 34*t*, 41*t*
Personal Experience Screening Questionnaire (PESQ), 64*t*
Personal problems, substance abuse and, 3
Person-centered approach to intervention, 165, 171–172
PESQ. *See* Personal Experience Screening Questionnaire
  (PESQ)
Pharmacotherapy, 99, 104
Phenobarbital, 46–48*t*
Planning
  consultation/referral and, 170–176
  crisis plans and, 186
  group interventions and, 147–151
  program implementation and, 85–91, 90*f*
Policy, school. *See* School policy
Poppers. *See* Nitrites
POSIT (Problem-Oriented Screening Instrument for
  Teenagers), 63–64, 64*t*, 67
Pregroup interviews, 152–153
Preschool, prevention programming and, 72
Pretreatment assessment, 111*t*, 113–114
Prevention groups, 131
Prevention programming
  case examples and, 91–93
  Drug Abuse Resistance Education Program (D.A.R.E.)
    evaluation and, 81–85
  implementation planning and, 85–91
  principles of drug abuse prevention and, 71–73
  program evaluation and, 73–81
  three levels of, 69–71, 70*f*
Privacy, 176. *See also* Confidentiality
Problem-Oriented Screening Instrument for Teenagers
  (POSIT), 63–64, 64*t*, 67
Problem-solving skills, group interventions and, 149–150*f*
Professionalization, of prevention programs, 89, 90*f*
Project Towards No Drug Abuse (TND), 75–77
Prosocial behaviors, individual interventions and, 106
Protective factors
  case examples and, 41*t*
  individual interventions and, 98–99
  prevention and, 71
  for substance abuse, 31–39, 34*t*
Psychoeducation groups, 131, 131*f*, 180–182, 181*t*, 187*f*
Psychostimulants, 3. *See also* Substance use
Purpose, group, defining, 149–150*f*

Quaalude, 46–48*t*, 50
Questioning skills, 140

Racial considerations
  case examples and, 158–160
  consultation/referral and, 165, 174–176
  group interventions and, 145–147

individual interventions and, 124
  lifetime prevalence rates and, 12*f*, 13*f*, 14*f*, 15*f*
  prevention and, 72
  rapport building and, 139–140
  rates of substance use and, 12–14
RAPI (Rutgers Alcohol Problem Index), 64*t*
Rapport building, 139–140
Readiness for program implementation, 88–91, 90*f*
Reconnecting Youth (RY), 77–79
Referral
  case examples and, 191–193
  coordination of treatment and, 186–188, 187*f*
  information gathering and, 170–176
  key features of, 164–166
  matching services and, 179–186
  needs identification and, 166–170
  overview of, 163–164
  resource location and, 177–179
  systemic process of, 189–191, 191*f*
Reinforcement of deviant behavior, group interventions
    and, 157–158
Relapse prevention plans, 109, 111*t*
Residential treatment settings, 99–100, 108*f*, 181*t*, 185–186,
    187*f*
Resistance, 115, 143–144
Resources, consultation/referral and, 177–179
Reward pathways, substance abuse and, 27
Risk factors
  case examples and, 41*t*
  collaboration and, 174
  continuum of substance use and, 181*t*
  individual interventions and, 98–99
  Student Screening Decision Sheet (SSDS) and, 60–62,
    61*f*
  for substance abuse, 31–39, 34*t*
Ritalin, 3, 46–48*t*, 51. *See also* Substance use
Rohypnol, 46–48*t*, 49, 52–53
Rutgers Alcohol Problem Index (RAPI), 64*t*
RY (Reconnecting Youth), 77–79

Sample Release of Information Form, 19*f*
SAPs (student assistance programs), 101
Scheduling considerations, group interventions and, 151–152
School factors
  individual interventions and, 106, 107–110, 108*f*
  problems with school and, 3
  risk/protective factors and, 34*t*, 37–38, 41*t*
  self-help groups and, 132–133
School policy
  consultation/referral and, 166
  existing policies and, 190–191, 191*f*
  group interventions and, 154
  individual interventions and, 96–97
  overview of, 1–2, 16
  screening and. *See* Screening
  zero tolerance as, 2, 16, 20–21, 39–42
School-based intervention settings, 100–101, 108*f*, 187*f*
Screening, 55–65, 61*f*. *See also* Assessment
Seconal, 46–48*t*
Selected prevention programs, 70–71, 70*f*. *See also* Three-
    tiered prevention programs

Selective seratonin reuptake inhibitors (SSRIs), 99
Self-awareness, group leaders and, 146
Self-efficacy expectations, substance abuse and, 30–31
Self-help groups, 131*f*
Self-management strategies, 180–182
Self-recording behavior, psychoeducation and, 180–182
Self-reinforcement, 180–182
Services, student, gaps in, 91
Settings, treatment, 99–101
Severity, problem, 86–88, 168
Size, group, 151
Social environment
    individual interventions and, 106, 111*t*
    pressures of, 163
    See also Family factors; Peer factors; School factors
Social learning theory, substance abuse and, 29–31
Socioeconomic status, 39, 65–67, 72, 174–175. *See also*
    Community factors
Solvents, 46–48*t*, 54
Sopor, 46–48*t*
Space considerations, group interventions and, 151–152
SSDS, 60–65
SSRIs (selective serotonin reuptake inhibitors), 99
Stabilization, of prevention programs, 89, 90*f*
Stages of group development, 133–138, 134*f*
Steroids, 7*f*, 8*f*, 9*f*. *See also* Substance use
Stimulants
    lifetime prevalence rates and, 11*f*, 14*f*, 15*f*
    substance abuse and, 46–48*t*, 50–51
    as substances, 3
    See also Substance use
Structure
    as aspect of prevention programs, 73–74
    Drug Abuse Resistance Education Program (D.A.R.E.)
        and, 83
    indicated prevention programs and, 77, 78
    three-tiered prevention programs and, 80
    universal prevention programs and, 75
Student assistance programs (SAPs), 101
Student population, substance use and, 10
Student Screening Decision Sheet (SSDS), 60–65, 61*f*
Student services, gaps in, 91
Students
    collaboration and, 170–173
    requests for help from, 169–170
Sublimaze, 46–48*t*
Substance abuse
    biologically based theories of, 26–28
    continuum of substance use and, 181*t*
    defined, 3, 4, 8–9, 8*f*
    prevention of. *See* Prevention programming
    reasons for, 25–26
    social learning theory and, 29–31
    types of substances and, 45–55
    See also Substance use
Substance dependence
    continuum of substance use and, 181*t*
    defined, 9–10
    lifetime prevalence rates and, 9*f*

Substance use
    continuum of, 181*t*
    defined, 2–3, 4
    legal considerations and. *See* Legal considerations
    prevalence of, 1–2, 5–10
    school policies and. *See* School policy
    See also Substance abuse
Sudden sniffing death, 54
Suggested Structure for Intervention Based upon MET and
    CBT, 111*t*
Suicidality, residential settings and, 99
Summarization skills, 140–142
Support groups, 131–132, 131*f*
Symptom, defined, 3–4
Syndrome, defined, 3–4
Systems of care, 164

Teachers, collaboration and, 169–170, 170–173
Team-based approach to treatment, 190
Temperament, risk factors and, 31
Termination stage of a group, 134*f*, 137–138, 149–150*f*
THC, 53
Therapy groups, 131*f*, 133
Three-tiered prevention programs, 69–71, 70*f*, 79–81
Time considerations, group interventions and, 151–152
TND (Project Towards No Drug Abuse), 75–77
Tobacco, 46–48*t*. *See also* Cigarettes
Tolerance, defined, 4–5
Tranquilizers, 7*f*, 8*f*, 9*f*, 11*f*, 14*f*, 15*f*. *See also* Substance use
Transition stage of a group, 134*f*, 136–137
Treatment
    continuum of options for, 178
    versus prevention, 69
    settings, 99–101
    See also Intervention
Treatment orientation, defined, 98
Trust, 58, 171
12-step model, 101–102. *See also* Alcoholics Anonymous
    (AA)
Twins, substance abuse and, 28

Understanding, mental health professionals and, 58
Universal prevention programs, 70–71, 70*f*, 74–75. *See also*
    Three-tiered prevention programs

Valium, 46–48*t*
Vicodin, 46–48*t*, 52

War on drugs, 20
Wellbutrin, 99
Withdrawal, 4–5, 27
Working stage of a group, 134*f*, 137
Workload, school professional's role and, 167–168
Wraparound approach, 164

Xanax, 46–48*t*

Zero tolerance policies, 2, 16, 20–21, 39–42
Zoloft, 99